FINDING & FUNDING

Residential Care for the Elderly

<small>FINDING & FUNDING</small>

Residential Care for the Elderly

<small>TERRY FRUIN</small>

**KOGAN
PAGE**

First published in 1995

Kogan Page Limited
120 Pentonville Road
London N1 9JN

© Terry Fruin 1995

British Library Cataloguing in Publication Data

A CIP record for this book is available from the British Library.

ISBN 0 7494 1312 3

Typeset by DP Photosetting, Aylesbury, Bucks
Printed and bound in Great Britain by
Clays Ltd, St Ives plc

Contents

Introduction

This book is designed to help those people who have identified a problem and in doing so have opened up a difficult process of decision making that is likely to become emotional, both for the individual, their family and close friends.

The problem relates to the ageing process and its effect on people who may no longer be able to cope with the many facets of day-to-day living, resulting in a decline in their quality of life and their need for care.

This self-help guide will take the reader through the intricacies of obtaining care for the elderly, with specific emphasis on residential care. It covers all aspects of the selection and provision of care and the organisation of various options; it lists the agencies, statutory, private and voluntary, that offer advice and assistance to all concerned. Addresses of these organisations are given in Chapter 6.

In the following chapters the various care options will be discussed with comments on any advantages and disadvantages. There is an explanation of the National Health Service and Community Care Act 1990 and an outline of people's 'right to care' under this Act. There is information covering the funding of various care options as well as details of statutory benefits, and suggestions for where to look, and whom to ask about the avail-ability of care. Also, there are checklists to help you consider the details of the various care options.

Throughout our lives we engage in forward planning

and, if we are honest, we realise that much of what happens to us results from plans laid down some time in the past. We plan our later education and careers, we plan which area of the social strata we prefer to be members of, and in this area we make friends, meet our prospective spouses and generally live our lives. We plan for short-term things like holidays. We plan our families and then our children's education. Then later we plan for our retirement in several ways, but always with the aim to provide a happy and meaningful life when we finish working.

Then a strange thing happens. In most cases we stop planning. Here we are at the crossroads of life, having reached retirement age, a time when all we have to look forward to is getting older and therefore less able to manage, and we stop planning for the future.

This book presents an opportunity to carry the planning process a stage further than just retirement. Perhaps now is the time to take on board the fact that ageing is a natural progression of life and that careful thought and financial provision now can lead to an even greater sense of achievement and peace of mind for many years to come.

It is hoped that the information in this book will help you to reach the correct decision about the type of care that you and your parents, relatives or close friends deserve. The final decision should be one that affords peace of mind to everyone concerned that an organised and comfortable care regime has been established, ensuring a high quality of life.

1. The Need for Care

Taking stock of your needs

As you grow older and are less able to manage the complexities of everyday life, it is necessary to take stock of your situation. This process can be a traumatic experience and requires a lot of soul-searching and honest appraisal of one's ability to cope safely and adequately about the home. The appraisal process can be further aggravated by not being aware of what care options exist and, more importantly, the financial implications of these options. Your main objective should be to achieve an environment that is easy to manage, is safe, warm and comfortable, and allows you to continue enjoying a full, independent and satisfactory way of life.

So, where should one start with this self-appraisal? Perhaps the best starting point is an honest assessment of your physical capabilities compared with, say, a year ago.

- Are you frailer now than you were then, and have you lost weight? If yes, how much?
- Are you less mobile?
- Is your eyesight deteriorating?
- Is your hearing as good as it was?
- Can you still manage steps and stairs?
- Do you have difficulty in reaching things, both at skirting board level or above your head?
- Are you losing your sense of smell?

- Are you becoming forgetful?
- Do you drop things frequently?
- Are you still able to get out and about?
- Can you still cook for yourself and make hot drinks?
- Do you still *like* cooking for yourself?
- Are you overreacting to a recent, and possibly temporary, problem?
- What does your GP say about your condition?

All the above questions relate to the process of ageing and may indicate that some form of care is needed. Now the problem lies not so much with the answers to your appraisal but in accepting those answers. All of us tend to feel much younger in mind than we are, but our physical appearance and prowess often tells another story.

Of course, it may be difficult to come to terms with the fact that you can no longer cope with all aspects of daily living on your own. Involving your family and friends in the process of what to do next could prove very helpful. It is likely that they may have been extremely concerned about your well-being over a long period, but have not known how to broach the subject. Furthermore, those family members that you do not see often may have noticed changes in your appearance and mobility that need to be considered. Once the matter of your need for care is out in the open, it ought to be possible for those closely involved to discuss the options rationally and effectively. Also, consultation within the family should prevent possible feelings of guilt and resentment cropping up in the future, particularly among younger relatives and friends. However, you should be aware that many conflicting feelings are involved.

The reluctance that many older people experience in deciding that care is essential is extremely common. Strong family ties can pose problems, not the least of

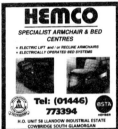
which can be a sense of failure and feelings of guilt on the part of the person needing care. There is also a possibility of conflicting opinions among family members and close friends as to whether care is needed, or what type of care would be of benefit. Often these conflicts can lead to a 'falling out' between people. The pressures that build up in a situation like this are in themselves difficult to come to terms with and inevitably add to the tension.

Beware of making emotional decisions. All too frequently close friends or family members are likely to say that you can move and live with them. Statements like: 'We'll look after you, don't worry' are all too common and come from the heart and not the head. They do demonstrate a caring attitude and stem from the love that others have for you. Inevitably, however, these offers have not been thought through.

It is important, therefore, that you try to keep control of the situation and retain a rational approach to the assessment process. Encourage those closely involved to discuss their views openly and constructively, and help you to reach the right decisions.

As an older person, your need for care may manifest itself in your being unable to cope with day-to-day activities within the home, with the result that your quality of life is greatly reduced.

You may be infirm and susceptible to falls – perhaps because your home is on more than one level and you have to climb stairs several times a day. Perhaps you have become very forgetful or confused which can pose problems of personal safety and security, and your home can be at risk in these situations. Although it is possible to set up some form of supervisory regime, it is virtually impossible to have a system that will ensure 24 hours of cover.

Yet another aspect to consider is loneliness, which in itself can present a different set of problems. While you might be physically capable and relatively alert mentally, the psychological effects of being alone can be extremely damaging. Often, this becomes evident through a deterioration in daily routines. There might be a tendency towards lapses in personal hygiene, and your home may not be cleaned as regularly or thoroughly as before. An attitude of not being bothered manifests itself which can result in your diet suffering and your going for long periods without adequate food. If you allow yourself to carry on in such a situation for too long, it is almost certain that you will develop physical infirmities and could become forgetful and confused.

The situations outlined above are generally a result of your getting old, and it is advisable to go and see your GP regularly so that he or she can keep an eye on your general condition. In any event, if any of the physical problems mentioned above persist for any length of time, you should certainly consult your GP.

When you discuss your need for care with those involved with your well-being, they are likely to experience a range of emotions and attitudes which may take you aback. Each person is likely to see your problem from a different perspective and react accordingly. Someone who visits you regularly is unlikely to notice any physical changes immediately, whereas one who visits less frequently will notice dramatic differences. Men are much less likely than women to notice any changes and therefore may react in a negative way to your need for care. However, any apparent lack of concern should not be seen as an uncaring attitude, it may be more a reluctance to accept the facts as they stand. You will be surprised by your own attitude and that of your family, once you make the difficult decision that you require care – how much more positive everyone, including you, becomes.

Now that your need for care is established and accepted, what are your options?

- Could you have your home adapted to make it more practical for your needs?
- Is a sheltered retirement home a prospect, either to rent or purchase?
- Could you go to live with a close friend or family member?
- Can an existing family dwelling have a 'granny flat' added?
- Is sheltered accommodation a possibility?
- Is a residential care home the only logical solution?
- What are the financial implications of the alternatives?
- How will the chosen option be funded?

Again, the practicalities of the various care options need to be investigated very carefully and some tough decisions taken. It is very important that your family and friends remain aware that any decision must be yours and must first of all suit your need. Although this may seem a selfish attitude, it is the only logical one. Once the decision is taken and a care regime installed, everyone will return to the daily lives that they enjoyed before the problem arose. *You* will be left with the consequences of the decision.

Having reached the end of the analysis and assessment process and come to a view as to the type of care that suits your needs, how do you go forward? The best way to proceed may be to visit your GP to inform him or her of the family's deliberations and of your decision. This would also be an opportunity to go over the physical and mental problems you have been experiencing and the effect these have had on your daily routines. You can also seek the doctor's advice about the viability of your choice and its long-term practicalities. At the same time the doctor can take note of your general physical and medical condition, and may give you a thorough examination. He or she will also be able to comment on your choice and may even suggest an alternative solution. At some stage in the future a report on your general medical condition will be required by the care assessor.

Another aspect of the community care initiative (as it has evolved after the implementation of the National Health Service and Community Care Act 1990) is that the medical profession seems to be redefining the concept of 'disability', and some doctors consider disability as a result of the ageing process. A person who is infirm and has difficulty in walking without an aid such as a walking stick is seen as being physically disabled, while someone who is forgetful or confused is deemed to have a sensory disability. The same applies to an elderly person whose eyesight is failing or who is hard of hearing.

The fundamental difference between current thinking and that of the past is that there is less of a stigma attached to being disabled. It is now recognised that a disabled person, irrespective of the type and level of disability, is entitled to care, help, information and education by right; also, that a person who is disabled has the right of choice in accepting this assistance or not. There is more detailed information about the right to care for disabled people in the section on pages 20–23.

So if you are deemed to be disabled due to the effects of ageing, try to be positive and accept the classification as a matter of fact. It does not make you any less of a person, it just says that here is someone who deserves to be cared for.

The assessment process

If you think that you need care, you have a *right* to be assessed by the Social Services Department of your local authority. Your local authority has a *duty* to assess your need for care if they consider that such a need exists (National Health Service and Community Care Act 1990).

On looking at these two statements, however, there appears to be a possible area of conflict. Several organisations hold the view that a local authority has a duty to assess 'only if they think there is a need for care' and that this constitutes a possible 'get out clause', ready to be used should the occasion arise. It is further thought that such an 'occasion' might be the lack of financial resources at some time in the future, even though the Act expressly forbids the use of 'lack of financial resources' as a reason for not performing an assessment.

In view of this situation, it is advisable that you seek advice from your doctor, and if it is agreed that you need a care assessment, then your application must be accompanied by a letter from your GP.

The actual assessment is carried out by a trained member of the Social Services Department who must listen to what you have to say and also take notice of what your carer considers your needs to be – that is, provided you have a carer. The care assessor is required to find out what you think your needs are and what you can and cannot do for yourself. He or she will also want to know what kind of help you would like to receive and whether you want to stay in your own home or not. The assessor should report back to the 'team leader', and a decision will then be made as to your actual need for care and at what level. Any decision must be taken with regard to all the facts to hand which will include a report from your GP. They are not allowed to disregard any information.

Some people involved

It is possible that during the assessment period you will be visited in your home by an occupational therapist who will determine the limits of your ability to cope 'adequately and safely within the home environment'. You may also be asked to attend a day centre at a nearby hospital, or another such place, for further specialist assessment. If during the assessment you are found to have a health or housing need, the assessor *must* contact the appropriate authorities and alert them to your requirements.

If a need for care is established, you will be allocated a care manager who will consult with you directly and formulate a care plan. The care plan will contain all the details of the care package required to ensure that all your needs are met. This package could include help to be provided in your own home, with all necessary aids, adaptations and care support; or the plan could recommend a place in a residential care or nursing home. You have a right to choose the care package you want.

Each local authority offers different kinds of help and support and has its own range of services. Each authority has a different way of charging for services and its own formula for deciding how much you will be required to pay. The amount you will be asked to pay, if any, will be decided by means testing, but if you have more than £8,000 (1994) in savings and capital you will be required to meet the full fees.

If the care assessor carries out his or her duties correctly, there ought not to be any questions asked concerning your financial status. The assessment is solely concerned with your need for care, and it is only after a need for care has been established and a plan formulated that the matter of cost is addressed.

Your rights

Of course, you do not have to be assessed by the Social Services Department. You can be completely independent and establish your care need by other means; your GP should be able to advise you about your options.

However, do bear in mind that you have a right to assessment and that it will be carried out by trained professionals and is free of charge. A written care plan must be submitted for your approval and the requirements of the plan carried through.

If you should disagree with the assessment results or are unhappy with the decision or the care package offered, you have the right to complain. Your first step in doing this should be to follow the local authority's complaints procedure which should have been made known to you at the time you were assessed. Wherever possible and whenever it is thought necessary, do seek expert advice.

Providers of community care

The NHS and Community Care Act 1990 charges that the statutory agencies who will provide and purchase community care services are: the local authority; the District Health Authority; and the Family Health Services Authority.

The Act further requires that these agencies operate after full consultation with, and with the full agreement of local voluntary organisations, including housing associations.

Each of the statutory agencies has its major areas of responsibility, as outlined below:

The local authority comprises the social services, housing, education, leisure and environmental health departments. It is the Social Services Department that leads the community care programme, and does this in direct consultation with all other departments.

The District Health Authority (DHA). Under the provisions of the Act these authorities have new and important responsibilities which include the assessment of the health needs of the residents within their sphere and the planning of future needs. The DHA purchases services by contract with providers (hospital and community health services) to ensure that needs are met. It must also ensure that *all* residents of the community have access to a range of high quality, value-for-money services.

The Family Health Service Authority (FHSA). The main objective of such an authority is to secure better health for the community it serves by:

- Assessing the needs of the communities, particularly children, the elderly and those from minority ethnic communities;
- Assisting family health service practitioners, GPs, dentists, community pharmacists, optometrists in their awareness of community needs;
- Ensuring that residents are kept fully aware of, and given access to, family health services.

Within this broad and somewhat confusing framework, the statutory agencies have the responsibility to provide care for the elderly. What can be even more confusing is that the Act specifies the services these agencies *must* provide and those that they *may* provide; and it is this distinction which determines your *right* to various services.

In practice it is the local authority that has become the prime mover in the application of community care legislation, through its Social Services Department. As a result, local authorities appear to be interpreting the more nebulous areas of the legislation to suit their particular needs. In view of this situation, it is most important that people seeking help and information about care understand their rights.

Your right to care

In making a balanced assessment of your care needs, it is important to be aware of the effect that current legislation will have on any choice that you might make.

Since April 1993 the NHS and Community Care Act 1990 has been in force, and the central objectives of this legislation are to develop good quality services that provide as normal a lifestyle as possible for people to live in the community.

Community care is the provision of help and support for people who are affected by problems of ageing, mental illness, sensory or physical disability; who have severe learning difficulties, have an alcohol or drug dependency, or are ill from HIV infection. Community care is designed to help, support and encourage people within these categories to live as independently as possible in their own homes or in 'homely' settings within the community. Care in the community is also charged with the support and protection of family life by maintaining and, where practical, improving independent lifestyles. An integral part of community care is the setting up of initiatives and support for carers (relatives, friends and neighbours) who already provide the greatest amount of support to elderly and disabled people.

The rights of disabled or elderly people

The main points to remember are that where a right to care exists, the local authority *must* provide a service because of its duty to do so as laid down in an Act of Parliament. Where an Act says that the local authority *may* do something, this represents a *power* to act, but does not confer any rights on someone who *may* receive a service.

The two Acts of Parliament which give disabled people the *right* to social services are: the Chronically Sick and Disabled Persons Act 1970 (CSDP) and the Disabled Persons (Services, Consultation and Representation) Act 1986.

In the case of the CSDP Act the local authority is required to provide certain services to individual chronically sick and disabled people who normally reside in its area. However, only if a local authority is satisfied that the services are necessary to meet the 'needs' of the person *must* it then supply such services.

The services include the provision of or assistance with the following:

- disability aids and equipment within the home;
- adaptations to the home;
- meals at home or elsewhere;
- getting a telephone or any special equipment to use a telephone;
- taking advantage of educational or recreational facilities both inside and outside the home, including transport to and from the facilities;
- provision of holidays.

Under the provisions of the 1986 Act, you may ask for your needs to be assessed; and, if needed, you *must* be provided with services under the provisions of the CSDP Act.

The term 'disabled' refers to 'persons who are blind, deaf or dumb, and other persons who are substantially and permanently handicapped by illness, injury or congenital deformity or who are suffering from a mental disorder within the terms of the Mental Health Act' (National Assistance Act 1948) and to 'people who are partially sighted or hard of hearing' (Circular LAC (93) 10).

Mental illness, described in law as mental disorder, is defined as 'mental illness, arrested or incomplete development of mind, psychopathic disorder and any other disorder or disability of mind' (Mental Health Act 1983).

The above definitions apply to disabled people of all ages who can be registered as disabled with their Social Services Department. If you feel that you might be disabled in one way or another, a letter from your GP should be sufficient for your name to be registered. However, it is not essential that you are registered disabled or handicapped in order to receive services under the CSDP Act. It is only necessary to fit the definition of disability.

Since April 1993 a local authority has had a *duty* to *any* person whom it considers may be in need of community care services to carry out an assessment of that person's need; after the assessment the local authority must decide whether the need calls for the provision of the relevant services.

If during the assessment, it becomes clear that you are disabled, the local authority must assess your needs under the CSDP Act and the assessment *must* be comprehensive and cover your need for all local authority services such as housing in addition to social services. You do not have to ask for this assessment to be done – it should happen as a matter of course; however, it might also be of benefit to state that you consider yourself to be disabled.

If a local authority is satisfied that you need services, it is *required* to tell you that it *must* supply the services. If the services fall within the scope of the CSDP Act, the local authority cannot use lack of resources as an excuse not to provide the services, nor can it put you on a waiting list which would cause excessive delay in the provision of services.

You also have a right to your needs being assessed strictly on merit; and a local authority cannot refuse a request to supply services on the grounds of predetermined policies which might discriminate between one category of disability and another. Each application for assessment for a need for care services must be treated separately and comprehensively in its own right.

Under the provisions of the CSDP Act, a local authority cannot withdraw a service provided for a disabled person unless it can show conclusively that the need for the service no longer exists due to a significant change in the recipient's condition, either socially, physically or mentally.

The Social Services Department *must* provide on request all relevant information about all of its services, as well as those provided by other departments within the local authority. It must also inform you of other services offered by voluntary or private agencies if it knows about them. Usually, a Social Services Department will have all of this information to hand and contained within its community care plan.

Local authorities have also been instructed to ensure that when a person has been assessed, 'a copy of the assessment of needs should normally be shared with the potential user' and that 'this record will normally be combined with a written care plan'.

If a carer feels that there are grounds for a disabled person's needs to be assessed, the local authority *must* act and at the same time it *must* take into account the ability of the carer to continue his or her role. Carers are also able to ask to be assessed separately in respect of their own needs.

If it is apparent that an elderly person is unable to decide for him or herself whether to be assessed, a carer can ask for the assessment to be carried out. Likewise, if a local authority considers that a person appears to be in need of community care service, it can conduct any assessment as deemed necessary.

Local authorities *must* give people who are disabled, and their carers, information regarding local schemes where they may be able to get help from an independent representative (advocate) in stating their needs.

Your right to other services
Local authorities have a *duty* to arrange residential

accommodation for people who 'by reason of age, illness, disability or any other circumstances are in need of care and attention, which is not otherwise available to them'. They also have a duty to 'provide temporary accommodation for persons who are in urgent need thereof in circumstances where the need for that accommodation could not reasonably have been foreseen', as well as a duty to make arrangements for prevention, care, and after-care for people with mental disorder.

Local authorities will find elderly people a place in one of their own homes or purchase care in a voluntary or private sector residential home. They can also purchase care for people in voluntary or private nursing homes once they have approval from the district health authority.

Once a local authority has assessed a person and has offered a place in a residential or nursing home, it *must* give the person the opportunity to have a place in a home of their own choosing (the 'preferred accommodation') subject to certain conditions which include:

- that the home is suitable for the assessed need;
- that a place is available;
- that the place does not cost the local authority more than it would normally pay.

A place in a more expensive home can be arranged if someone other than the local authority is willing to make up the difference.

Services that may be provided

There are some services that a local authority has the *power* to provide but not a *duty* to do so. Therefore, when you see lists of local authority services that *may* be provided, do not assume that they *will* be provided. Likewise, you have no right of appeal if you are assessed as being in need of a service but the local authority has no funds available to supply it.

Services that a local authority *may* offer to disabled people include:

- Social work support and advice;
- Facilities at centres for social rehabilitation and adjustment;
- Facilities for occupational activities;
- Holiday homes;
- Provision of free or subsidised travel for those who do not qualify for travel concessions where such concessions are available;
- Assistance in finding suitable accommodation;
- Contribution towards the cost of employing a warden on welfare functions or providing welfare services in private housing.

Services a local authority *may* provide for *elderly but not disabled* people include the following:

- Meals and recreation in the home and elsewhere;
- Information about available services;
- Transport to and from a service provided by the authority or a voluntary agency;
- Assistance in finding suitable households for boarding out;
- Visiting and social work support;
- Practical assistance in the home (adaptations for safety, comfort or convenience).

Other services that a local authority *may* offer are:

- Meals on wheels;
- Night sitting services;
- Recuperative holidays;
- Facilities for social and recreational activities.

Carers' rights

As a carer you are allowed to act on behalf of someone who is elderly and frail, and unable to represent themselves adequately. You can make representation to the person's GP and seek an assessment of care needs from the local authority. It must be clearly understood that you cannot make a person do anything against their wishes. It should also be apparent to those concerned that you are acting in your charge's best interests. It is almost certain that the person's doctor and any social workers involved would want to assure themselves of this fact before proceeding.

Once your credibility is established you have the right within the law to act for the person for whom you care and are able to seek an assessment of their needs. You also have the right within the law to have your own needs assessed at the same time.

Perhaps the person you are caring for, who could be a relative or a friend, has become very frail, is perhaps a stroke victim or suffers from senile dementia or some similar condition. In such cases it is likely that the person being cared for is too frail to qualify for standard residential care but is not considered ill enough to qualify for nursing home care. As a result, you might experience great difficulty in finding a place for the person. If this is the situation, you should insist on an assessment being carried out by the local authority. As mentioned elsewhere, if the person is assessed as needing care, the local authority has a *duty* to provide the care and will *have* to find the person a place in a suitable home.

The person you care for might be in hospital and about to be discharged, and you may be unhappy about this. It is now customary for hospitals to discharge a patient once the medical staff feel that there is no more treatment from which the patient may benefit and if the patient's bed is needed for another admission. The decision to discharge a person is made on the basis of a clinical appraisal by a consultant. As a carer or a patient, you may be unhappy with this decision; and if so you should seek an appointment with the consultant and express your concern. You should state clearly and firmly, in writing if necessary, why you feel the discharge to be inappropriate.

As a carer, you should also resist any pressure to have the person moved from the hospital if there is no suitable alternative accommodation available. It is incumbent upon all hospitals to have proper discharge procedures that are lawful. If the person you care for has been assessed as needing continuous nursing care, they cannot be forced to move to a nursing or residential home against their wishes.

No one should feel forced to care for someone if this is not practicable or feasible, nor should anyone be forced to carry out the role of carer.

Appealing against the assessment

There is no right of appeal against the financial assessment carried out by a local authority. Should you wish to challenge the outcome of such an assessment, you will have to go through their complaints procedures.

If the points at issue cannot be resolved informally between the parties involved, and a satisfactory outcome achieved, you should proceed as follows:

- Make a 'formal registration' of your complaint in writing.
- The local authority should consider and respond within 28 days of its receipt.

- Failing this, they must give an explanation of the position within the first 28 days, and a full response within three months.
- You can request a review if you are not satisfied with their response and you must request this within 28 days.
- Within 28 days of receipt of the request for a review, a panel consisting of three people (one of whom must be independent of the local authority) should hold a meeting.
- You, as the complainant, must be given ten days' notice of the meeting, and the notice must include information about the time and place where the review is to be held and the name and status of the panel members.
- You must also be informed of your right to attend with another person, but *not* a solicitor or barrister acting in a professional capacity.
- The outcome of the review must be recorded within 24 hours and both sides must be notified in writing of the recommendations.
- The local authority will then have 28 days to decide on their course of action, if any, and they must inform you of the reasons for their decisions.

Appeals and complaints procedures

You have a right to complain if the local authority has not assessed you as being in need of a service, but you believe that you do require it, or you do not like the service or services being offered. The local authority *must* have a formal complaints procedure in place which must be explained to you in full. (Your right to complain is incorporated in the Local Authority Social

Services Act 1970 – section 7B as defined in section 50 of the National Health Service and Community Care Act 1990.)

If you do not get satisfaction through the local authority's complaints procedures and feel there has been a case of maladministration, you can approach the local government Ombudsman. Maladministration covers faults in the way in which things have been done and it may include neglect, discrimination, unjustified delay, failure to follow agreed procedures, or indeed not to have proper procedures. You may complain directly or through a local councillor, but you must make your complaint within 12 months of needing a service. The Ombudsman's investigations can take a long time and you should be aware that any recommendations made by the Ombudsman are not binding and that the local authority can choose to ignore them. However, the Ombudsman's report will be published.

The address of the relevant Ombudsman can be obtained from your local authority, a library or the Citizens' Advice Bureau.

You have the right of appeal to the Secretary of State for Health if you think that a local authority has a duty to provide a service but refuses to do so or withdraws a service or services. You, or someone acting for you, can report the local authority to the Secretary of State for Health who, in turn, may make an order declaring a local authority to be in default in respect of a duty if the Secretary of State is satisfied that the local authority has failed, without reasonable excuse, to comply with any of its duties which are social services functions. Any decision by the Secretary of State does not have to be made public; however, the local authority and the complainant will be informed.

Before making an appeal to the Secretary of State for

Health you should have been through the local authority's complaints procedures.

You could of course pursue the matter through the courts, in which case it would be advisable to consult a solicitor. At the same time you could also explore your eligibility for legal aid. You can sue the local authority for a breach of its statutory duty in which case you must be able to demonstrate the following:

- A specific need for which a service should be provided;
- Which service is required to satisfy such need;
- That you have requested the service;
- The local authority has failed to satisfy the need.

It is likely that court action will be very time consuming, frustrating, and the case difficult to prove. Another avenue would be to seek a *judicial review* of the local authority's actions in the High Court, in which the court can be asked to examine whether the local authority's actions have been *legal, rational, and reasonable.* The main grounds for challenge are:

- Illegality: that the local authority got the law wrong.
- Irrationality: the local authority has acted in an unreasonable manner in making a decision.
- Procedural impropriety: the local authority has failed to follow correct procedures and to take into account all relevant considerations, including representation from the affected person.

The court is not allowed to substitute its own views for those of the decision-making authority, but it does have the power to set aside any decision on the grounds that the local authority acted improperly in reaching the said decision. At this stage the matter is then referred back to the local authority for a new decision.

The procedure for applying for a judicial review has two stages:

1. An application is made for leave to apply for a judicial review; then
2. If leave is granted the case will proceed and be heard.

Local authorities have been known to reconsider and reverse decisions under threat of this type of court action, especially at the stage when leave is granted to apply for judicial review.

Summary

As you can see from the above information the whole subject of care can be confusing and difficult. However, once you grasp the difference between a local authority's *duty* and its *powers* under the various Acts, the situation may become somewhat clearer. It is always advantageous to understand your rights when talking to local authority officials. If you are unsure about any aspect of your right to care or services, do seek expert advice from the Community Health Council or your local Citizens' Advice Bureau.

2. Exploring the Care Options

Gathering information on the care options available is time consuming and can be quite frustrating. Since the NHS and Community Care Act 1990 came into force, the task has become somewhat more daunting because you now have to deal with officials and jargon. This chapter covers the main care options available to elderly people, what each option entails and its advantages and possible disadvantages. Also mentioned are various agencies, private, voluntary and statutory, that offer advice, information and assistance within these options. However, do note that the inclusion of any agency, particularly a commercial one, is in no way a recommendation. In exploring the options for care, you must ask all the questions and draw your own conclusions.

Staying at home

Current legislation makes it plain that the government's wish is that elderly people requiring care should be supported in their own homes for as long as is practical. In response to this wish local authorities have contingency plans to provide care in the community, though it is likely to differ from one council to another.

Each authority will also have its own way of costing these services and deciding how much you will have to pay. The Social Services Department of your local authority should furnish details of the services provided for community care, but do ask other organisations what should be available. A chat with your local councillor might also be helpful.

The main area to consider with regard to this option is how you can best adapt, modify or improve your home to make it more manageable. An objective assessment of your home and its facilities should be undertaken and preferably with the assistance of someone experienced in these matters. Perhaps you should make a list headed 'Aids' and 'Adaptations' and make notes for future reference and discussion. Here are some points you will want to consider:

- Are there steps to the front of the house or apartment block?

- Could they be replaced by a gently sloping ramp?
- Is the front door wide enough to take a wheelchair if necessary?
- Is there a step into the doorway; should this be taken out?
- Is the keyhole easily reachable?
- Does the entrance hall have adequate space for manoeuvring a wheelchair or walking frame? Are other door frames wide enough?
- Are light switches and power points accessible?
- Are the stairs manageable; is there a grab rail as well as the bannister?
- Would a stair lift be more suitable?
- Do water taps need to be replaced with those of a better design?
- Are there adequate heating arrangements?
- Is there any heavy and cumbersome furniture making mobility difficult?
- Does the back door need widening or re-siting?
- Are there steps to the garden that could be replaced with a ramp?
- Do the window catches need replacing?
- Are any major repairs needed?

There are probably many more items to add to your list, but the main point to remember is that your final question should be 'When all these alterations have been done, will I be able to manage, safely and comfortably?'

Aids for daily living are usually recognised as being gadgets or equipment designed to help you if you have a problem managing certain tasks. They can include amplifiers for telephones and televisions, magnifiers for partially sighted people, and gadgets to help you get out of bed and dress. The list seems endless but an occupational therapist from the Social Services Department should be able to tell you what aids you might find helpful. The Disabled Living Foundation and the Disabled Living Centres Council are other useful sources of information. Some aids may be available on loan from the Red Cross, your local Age Concern, the WRVS (Women's Royal Voluntary Service), or the Carers' National Association.

After your home has been adapted, there may be other areas where the local authority can offer help and support. All services come under the auspices of community care and the local authority has the *power* to supply them, but not a *duty* to do so, unless you are disabled.

Alarm systems

Some elderly people who live alone have a greater feeling of security if their home is linked to an alarm system that enables them to contact a central bureau in an emergency. There are many different types of personal alarm, some of which can be supplied by local authority housing or social services departments. Others are offered by private companies.

Further information on alarm systems and suppliers can be obtained from the Disabled Living Foundation and Help the Aged (Community Alarms Department).

Day care

Several kinds of community day care are available and offer a chance to meet other people and perhaps share in activities and a meal. Some day-care centres offer special facilities to those suffering from disabling conditions and may also provide services at weekends. For people who are looked after by a carer who goes out to work, there are 'long' day-care centres; and some rural areas even have mobile centres. You will need to ask what is available in your community; and if you feel that a particular service or kind of care is required, you should ask whether it might be provided.

Home care assistant (home help)

Although home helps have long provided assistance in the home with cleaning, shopping and other practical tasks, some local authorities are no longer offering this service. Instead they now offer a new and more targeted service, providing more specialised care to those most in need. As a result of this shift in emphasis, organisations such as Age Concern now work closely with local authorities to set up home care schemes. In some areas private agencies offer help at home, but this can be quite costly. The Crossroads Care Attendant Scheme, which offers regular help in order to relieve carers, may run a service in your area. For information about private home care, contact the United Kingdom Home Care Association.

Laundry services

A few social services departments provide laundry services for people who are incontinent or cannot manage to do their own laundry for various reasons. As local authority provision is scarce, you may want to look in the *Yellow Pages* for local laundry services to contact.

Meals on wheels

There are several different kinds of meals on wheels services, and what you receive will depend on your needs and the policy of the local authority. There may be provision for people on special diets. Some meal services are run by Age Concern and the WRVS for councils. Some agencies provide a freezer for people to have at home and then deliver frozen meals so that they can heat their food when they so wish. Meals can be delivered on any number of days in the week. There is usually a nominal charge for the service, though in some circumstances this may be waived.

Respite care

Respite care is often available to provide a break for both the carer and the person being cared for. This respite could be for a night or a day or a longer period, say, a week or two. In some areas it is possible to arrange such care in the person's home, but more usually respite care is provided in residential care, nursing homes or hospitals.

Sitting-in schemes

There are 'sitting-in' schemes run by social services departments and other organisations, designed to give carers a break. It can be arranged for someone to 'sit in' an older person's home on a regular basis or only in the case of an emergency.

Telephones

If you need to have a telephone installed, you may be able to get help with meeting the costs from your local Social Services Department. Some charities may also offer help. British Telecom offers information and advice on adaptions and equipment if you are having difficulty in handling their standard systems.

Live-in companions

Some elderly people may prefer to have a live-in companion in their home because of the added feeling of security such an arrangement might offer. They probably feel that a companion could keep a watchful eye on them, assist around the house with light housework, and undertake other tasks that could be agreed.

Anyone seeking a live-in companion should exercise

extreme caution when selecting a likely candidate and should ask for references. The wording of any advertisement should be drafted very carefully and all replies directed to a box number. It would be a good idea to list all the tasks you would expect the person to perform and obtain written acceptance of such a 'job description' from the successful applicant. Advice should be sought on such things as salary, income tax and National Insurance contributions, as these must be met and accounted for. Perhaps a contract of employment should be drawn up and other safeguards introduced.

A number of private agencies exist who recruit and place live-in companions, day or longer-term nurses and care workers. It is essential that you specify exactly what you expect from such an arrangement and assess whether the service being offered will actually meet your requirements. Each agency is likely to operate differently and their charges will reflect this difference.

For further information refer to the *Yellow Pages* for names of employment agencies and private nursing agencies. Other organisations offering help and advice are: the United Kingdom Home Care Association and Counsel and Care for the Elderly.

The advantages of staying put are obvious. You remain in your home surroundings in which there is already a history of occupancy and a sense of belonging. You are known in the locality by neighbours, friends, shopkeepers and others, and your family and relatives also know, and are comfortable with, your environment. You retain a high level of independence.

The disadvantages may occur at some future time when, perhaps you become less mobile, loneliness may become a factor and you could become reclusive.

Staying put is a choice only you can make.

Sheltered retirement homes

There are different kinds of sheltered housing schemes available to rent or buy. Generally speaking, they range from simple bed-sit accommodation to luxury apartments. All good schemes will have an alarm system, be warden controlled and have communal facilities, but the level and quality of these facilities can be variable.

Whether you rent or buy one of these properties, it should conform to a minimum design standard and some of the things to look for are listed below:

- Is the emergency alarm system linked to the warden and to a 24-hour monitoring service?
- Is the sheltered scheme on more than one floor, and are apartments above the ground floor accessible by stairs or lifts?
- Are doorways and corridors within the unit you are considering wide enough to accommodate walking frames and wheelchairs?
- Do the doors and windows have handles and catches that are easy to operate?
- Are the light switches and power points accessible without the need for bending and stretching?
- Are the rooms adequately heated and by what means? Is there ample ventilation?
- Is the apartment or house well insulated against noise? Check for sounds coming from adjoining properties.
- Is there an excess of outside noise from lifts, communal doors opening and closing or from the communal rooms or the laundry?
- Are the rooms in the unit you are considering large enough to house your furniture and belongings, or will you need to dispose of some items?
- Are there facilities for accommodating guests?
- Is there adequate parking space for visitors?

After establishing the quality of design, the next important area to investigate is the management of the complex, with particular regard to charges, and the duties of the warden.

The warden's duties

Most sheltered housing projects have a resident warden; a few, however, may have a person who carries out the duties of a warden but does not live on the site.

It is important to find out how many hours in the day the warden is on duty, and what arrangements for cover are made when he or she is off duty. It is unusual to have 24-hour cover, so it will be necessary to learn what relief facilities are in place. The duties of a warden are usually those of a 'good neighbour', someone who keeps a watchful eye on the residents. Some wardens help out with shopping and getting prescriptions filled, although this is the exception rather than the rule. It is essential that you get a written and concise description of the warden's duties from the project managers. This can save confusion and disappointment at a later stage; it will also provide you with a means of checking on the level and quality of service that you actually receive. It is a fact that the warden's salary and employment costs will form a large proportion of the service charge levied.

Whether renting or buying, it is vital that any contract offered to you is looked at and vetted by your solicitor, also that you are fully aware of your obligations.

Renting a sheltered retirement home

There are numerous organisations that offer sheltered accommodation for rent and, generally speaking, they fall within the categories already described. The main provider of such properties is likely to be your local authority; however, several organisations work closely with local councils to provide, or advise on, this type of housing. They are, in the main, housing associations and charitable trusts some of which are mentioned below.

- National Federation of Housing Associations
- The Housing Corporation
- HOMES (Housing Organisations Mobility and Exchange Services)
- English Churches Housing Group
- Elderly Accommodation Counsel

A fuller list of housing associations can be found in Chapter 6.

Buying a sheltered retirement home

If you are contemplating buying one of these homes, you will need to exercise caution and seek expert legal advice. Usually, sheltered housing is accommodation in a group of self-contained flats, sometimes bungalows, situated within a purpose-built development. Generally, the properties are put up by a builder and the freehold is held by a management service company.

The properties are usually sold on a long lease and only to people aged 55 or over. The management company runs the complex on a day-to-day basis, taking care of all communal areas and gardens, maintaining and repairing where necessary. The management also employs the resident warden, if there is one. For these services, they levy an annual management fee payable by all households. Historically, there have been numerous occasions where residents have been unhappy with the service provided and fees charged. In order to address these problems and allay the fears of prospective buyers, the industry now has two main regulatory bodies which offer various safeguards. They are the Association of Retirement Housing Managers and the National House

Building Council (NHBC). Both these organisations operate a code of practice.

The NHBC concerns itself with the companies that build and develop sheltered housing and offers a new-home warranty called 'Buildmark'. The NHBC has introduced a code of practice (a copy of which is available on request, at a nominal charge) which requires that its registered members must ensure that residents' rights are fully protected by a legally binding management agreement between themselves and the management organisation. The code is applicable to all sheltered housing built and sold or let by an NHBC member after 1 April 1990. If the housing project was built before April 1990 the builder and management organisation should give purchasers as many as possible of the rights named in the code.

The code also states that when a potential buyer has paid a reservation fee, the builder must provide a Purchaser's Information Pack which must include detailed information of numerous aspects of the purchase, including the following main points:

- The name and address of both the builder and the management organisation, details of any relationship between the two parties and whether the management organisation has an 'interest' in the lease.
- An undertaking by the management organisation that it will enter into a legally binding obligation with each purchaser to meet the requirements of the code of practice.
- Details of your legal rights as the purchaser, about the type of lease, service charges and the insurance arrangements; your right to be consulted about repairs, your rights if the management organisation fails to deliver any services agreed, and your rights if you should become frail or ill.

- A full and clear description of all facilities and services provided by the management organisation, which should include details of the alarm system. The warden's duties and hours of work must be clearly defined and stated, as must details of emergency and relief cover.
- A comprehensive, clear and detailed explanation must be furnished as to how the responsibilities for repairs will be divided between the builder, the management and the resident. The procedure for reporting repairs must also be clearly defined.
- Insurance details in respect of the buildings and contents of the communal areas must be made known to the resident.
- Full details of all payments, fees or charges that the resident is liable to pay to the house builder or management organisation.
- A full and detailed explanation of the way in which all the services are to be charged and how these charges will be apportioned between the dwellings.
- An explanation of the 'sinking fund' for long-term major repairs and redecoration, how it will be funded and what it will cover.
- A detailed explanation of the conditions for reselling including details of charges made by the management organisation when a property is sold.
- The lease, or management deed if the purchase is freehold. It is vital that this document is handed to a solicitor for safe keeping as soon as it is received.

Other sheltered housing schemes

Most sheltered housing is sold at full market value, and you get back the full value when you sell, less any retention or charges made by the management organisation. There are other schemes, however, which are worth consideration; but once again *do seek professional advice* before making a decision or signing an agreement. These other schemes include the following:

- With a *shared ownership* scheme, you may buy a share of the sheltered housing and pay rent on the remainder. A shared ownership scheme may be operated by a local authority and a housing association. A call to the regional office of the Housing Corporation should get you details of shared ownership properties in your area.

- *Leasehold schemes for the elderly (LSEs).* There are a few housing associations running this sort of scheme, whereby you buy 70 per cent of the lease with the balance funded by Housing Corporation subsidy. If you sell or leave you receive 70 per cent of the value realised.

- Some developers may offer a property at a discounted purchase price. Obviously, this will affect the amount you receive when you sell, but it should never be less than the discounted percentage.

- Other developers offer purchase options through a finance company at a percentage of the asking price. The older you are, the less you will pay, but when you die, the entire value of the property passes to the finance company.

- Ownership by a younger relative is usually allowed, but only people of 55 years and over may take up residency. This type of purchase can be very complicated, and expert legal advice is imperative.

Summary

The advantages of living in a sheltered retirement home are numerous, and provided you are happy with the arrangements and legalities, such a move could be extremely rewarding. The downside is that you will be living in an environment populated by elderly people. You will see the same faces day in, day out, and this could become tiresome and depressing. Another aspect is the question of service charges; experience shows that they are likely to increase year by year. Before making a decision, be sure you can afford it in the long term.

Other living arrangements

Living with a friend or family member

This option is by far the most popular with the statutory agencies because it is the most cost effective. It is likely that local authority representatives will try to persuade you and your carers that this option would be your best choice. They may very well be right, but the deciding factor should be how well you and your family get on together. It is important to put sentiment to one side and take a dispassionate look at what is involved. Remember that you are looking at a way of life that could continue over a long time span and will be completely different from a temporary stay of a few weeks or months. Will you and the prospective carer be compatible, and remain so, over a long period? You and your friend or family should know each other very well and should be honest with each other in the discussions that are bound to take place about whether you should live with a family member. It is better, perhaps, to hurt someone's feelings now by being frank rather than spending several years in difficult circumstances by not being honest.

Where is the care to take place? If it is to be in your home, will the prospective carer adapt to the change? Is the house suitable to take an extra occupant? The most important factor to keep in mind is that we all grow old together, and as you age so will your carer. What will happen to you if your carer becomes ill or unable to cope?

If the care is to take place in someone else's home, what will you do with yours? Is there sufficient room in the new environment to house you comfortably? What will the family have to sacrifice to make room for you? Present-day housing is not usually designed to accommodate an elderly person in an established household. Children have been encouraged to expect their own bedrooms, a private space in which they can develop. Do we expect them to give up this privacy to cater for granny or grandpa? The family unit has generally become outward looking in its everyday life, while the pressure of working and keeping house and home together has become the responsibility of both parents. All these contributing factors combine to make the traditional method of caring for an older person an extremely difficult undertaking.

Although the prospect of being cared for by a close friend or your family may appear attractive from an emotional standpoint, your main difficulty is going to be in making your decision a practical one.

Some people have their houses extended to make a small apartment or a garage converted into a self-contained bedsitting-room. The resulting living space or 'granny flat' may be an alternative worth considering. The main advantage is that both parties in the arrangement retain a high level of independence, but there remains an element of supervision and care. It would seem that local authorities are looking sympathetically at planning applications for granny flats, and of course there is the possibility that the plans might attract grants. The cost implications of building a granny flat are quite extensive, and there would be tremendous upheaval while the building work is being carried out. Careful thought and planning is essential with such a project, and of course, expert advice.

Sheltered accommodation

Not to be confused with sheltered housing, this care option usually consists of bedsit accommodation within a larger house, offering 24-hour supervision. Residents are encouraged to furnish their own rooms where possible, and can take their meals separately or communally. This type of accommodation is not widely available, and the projects are often run by charitable trusts, church charities and other similar organisations. The advantage of this option is that you are encouraged to have your possessions about you and retain a high level of independence. The organisations which provide sheltered accommodation work closely with local charities as well as the local authority. Much of their work is carried out by volunteers from all walks of life, and as a result the service they give covers a wide range of skills.

Some organisations active in providing sheltered accommodation and offering help with advice and information are:

- Abbeyfield Society
- Almshouse Association
- Country Houses Association Ltd
- Elderly Accommodation Counsel
- English Churches Housing Group
- English Courtyard Association
- Friends of the Elderly and Gentlefolk's Help
- Guild for Aid for Gentlepeople
- The Guinness Trust
- Help the Aged (Help the Aged – Gifted Housing Scheme)

- Homelife/Distressed Gentlefolk's Aid Association
- Jewish Care
- Methodist Homes for the Aged
- North British Housing Association Group
- Northern Ireland Housing Executive
- Presbyterian Housing Association (NI) Ltd
- Quaker Social Responsibility and Education

Home-from-Home schemes

Home-from-Home began in Liverpool and Leeds some ten years ago, and since that time has grown so that there are now nearly 250 schemes operating nationwide.

The schemes offer an alternative to the more conventional forms of residential care in that they provide a type of adult fostering arrangement. Elderly people who must give up their homes because they can no longer cope with looking after themselves are matched with host families and are given care and attention as if they were a member of the host family.

The objectives of the scheme are: 'To extend the current range of services offered to the elderly, by creating a new resource and thereby introducing an element of consumer choice.' In addition, there is the objective 'to provide a service of high quality that gives a completely tailored form of care and attention, designed to meet individual needs.'

Further details about Home-from-Home schemes are available from: The Secretary, Special Interest Group – Adult Placement Schemes (address page 149).

A useful source of further information on managing your financial affairs is: *Good Retirement Guide 1995* by Rosemary Brown, published by Kogan Page.

3. Residential and Nursing Home Care

Moving into a residential care home is an enormous step which should not be taken without a great deal of thought, and only after a thorough investigation of the alternatives. You should also discuss the matter fully with family and friends, and seek advice from as many knowledgeable sources as possible.

Making the decision

The reasons for choosing the care-home option can be varied, but the main ones are security, companionship and an inability to cope on a day-to-day basis.

Security. You may feel insecure in your home environment, particularly in the absence of 24-hour care, and although you may have an alarm system installed, you feel vulnerable when the carer leaves and you are left alone. It is likely that you will be on your own for up to 12 hours. What happens if you have a fall or become unwell during this time? It is not uncommon for imagined situations like these to cause extreme anxiety which in turn can lead to other complications. In such circumstances residential care could be the answer.

Companionship. Perhaps you have no close family and your circle of friends has diminished due to ill health or death. You may be quite fit and relatively active but problems of loneliness are becoming more apparent. Moving to a residential care home could solve this problem through the companionship of the other residents. The fact that the care home will take responsibility for providing food and drink and other essentials would probably allow you more free time to develop other active interests.

Inability to cope. It may be that the care package and support you receive in your own home is no longer suited to current needs. Perhaps your carer can no longer cope and the support services have become inadequate as a result. It could be that you now have mobility problems, perhaps your eyesight is failing or you are suffering from some other ageing disability. Whatever the reason, it is probably true to say that your quality of life has deteriorated and your day-to-day existence is becoming very stressful. In such a situation residential care may be the only logical solution.

However, no matter what your reasons are, you should take your time and give the matter a lot of careful consideration.

What is involved?

You might like to give some thought to the following list of consequences of moving to a care home:

- The move will probably be permanent.
- Such a move will mean disposing of your home, furniture, and most of your possessions.
- Your living space in a residential home will be limited, at best a bedsitting-room, but more likely a bedroom – and will involve sharing communal facilities such as residents' lounges and dining rooms; as a consequence

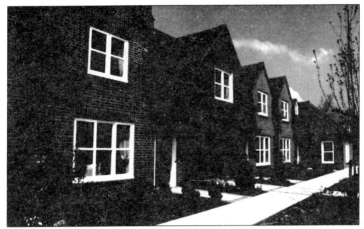

CHURCH PLACE, ICKENHAM, MIDDLESEX

A superb development of 25 large cottages and apartments on the very edge of London where much of the village atmosphere remains. The village pump, the pond, the 14th century church of St Giles, the Coach and Horses and the ancient Home Farmhouse are the setting for Church Place. There are excellent shops and facilities just across the road. Access to Central London is very easy via the Piccadilly, Metropolitan or Central lines and also to major routes out of London by way of the M40, M4 or M25 motorways.

English Courtyard Association remain leaders in their own field, achieving over 30 awards and commendations since their first site in 1977.

YOU KNOW WHAT YOU WANT WHEN YOU RETIRE.
Find it with us.

- ◼ We build superb properties for older buyers all over the country.
- ◼ Cottages and apartments, set in beautiful gardens, designed for comfort and security, ease and independence.
- ◼ Prices from £95,000 - £230,000. Each with its own garage.

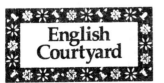
English Courtyard

For further information please contact us at:-
8 Holland Street, London W8 4LT.
FREEFONE 0800 220858.

there is likely to be little space to house many of your belongings.
- You may not be allowed to keep a pet.
- It is unlikely that the home will be situated in your own neighbourhood.
- As a result of this, friends and neighbours might not visit too often, and it could lead to a tailing off of their visits in the long term.
- You could experience some resentment from family and friends, particularly if they have not been party to your decision.
- There will be an inevitable loss of some of your independence.
- There is bound to be an element of regimentation in the daily routine of the home.

The biggest problem you are likely to face during this period is that of coming to terms with your need for residential care and accepting this as fact. Once you accept this need you will probably find your whole outlook becoming more positive and you will approach the next stage with confidence. If, however, you are still not 100 per cent sure about residential care, give consideration to a trial stay at a home; most establishments offer places on trial for up to a month, sometimes longer.

Whatever you decide to do, remember that no one can make you do anything you do not want to. You must do what is best for your own needs.

When you finally decide that residential care is your best option, what next?

Finding the right kind of home

Registered homes

There are three main categories of residential care homes – local authority, voluntary and private – and under the

Registered Homes Act 1984 all private and voluntary residential homes with four or more residents *must* register with the local authority. The Registration and Inspection Unit of the Social Services Department of a local authority must inspect all homes at least twice each year and the certificate of registration must be prominently displayed in the home. Private and voluntary residential homes having fewer than four residents are required to register with the local authority as a 'small home'. The registration procedure requires that the person running the home is deemed a 'fit person' to do so.

It follows that a local authority care home will automatically comply with the requirements of the Registered Homes Act 1984.

What constitutes a residential home?

A residential home is one in which the residents will receive full board and personal care to an agreed standard. It is likely that the level of care will vary from home to home. The Department of Health has defined the level of care as being that which would be given by a competent caring relative. This includes help with washing, bathing, toilet needs, dressing and eating, also nursing care in the case of illness at the same level that a family would provide in a similar situation. However, residential care does not include constant nursing care. As a result, some residential homes may not accept people with certain conditions. These are likely to include incontinence, mental health problems, learning disabilities, mild or severe confusion, Alzheimer's disease, multiple sclerosis, diabetes, or epilepsy. Other homes will be registered to provide care for specific conditions or may in fact have *dual registration*; that is, they will be registered as a nursing home with the District Health Authority as well as a residential home with the local council.

Contracts

If the local authority arranges for your placement in a registered care home they must ensure that they get the best possible care for you at the best price. A contract should therefore be drawn up between themselves and the care provider, and the said contract must contain all the requirements in your care plan. You should be allowed to verify this for yourself with the local authority. The contract should state the financial terms and the way in which the fee is payable. Either the local authority will pay the whole fee and collect your contribution and that of a third party where necessary; or you will pay your contribution directly to the home and the council, and a third party when applicable will pay their contribution separately to the home.

Local authority care homes

Some residential care homes are run by the local Social Services Department; known in some quarters as 'council care homes' they are becoming something of a rare commodity. With the constant financial constraints placed on local authorities over recent years, the trend is for them to 'purchase' residential care services from the voluntary and private sectors. As a consequence, many council (local authority) establishments are being closed. However, your own council may have facilities still operating and it is always worth asking what is available. Contact your local Social Services Department.

Voluntary organisation homes

These homes are usually run on a non-profit basis by charitable organisations, church groups, benevolent associations and other similar bodies. It is likely that admission to one of these homes would be subject to certain conditions such as past membership of a trade union, a trade or profession, perhaps a religious association, while in some cases admission may be exclusive to residents of a particular area. If you feel that you meet some of these special requirements, then this type of home might be just what you are looking for.

Private homes
In this category are those homes owned and run by private individuals, partnerships or companies. The main criterion is that they are all profit-seeking organisations, but this does not mean that the homes are run any less professionally. It is unlikely that a private residential home will have many conditions of acceptance, except perhaps the suitability of the resident to live in a particular home. Because it is geared to making profit, such a home will probably keep strictly to the contents of an agreed care plan. In view of this it is advisable to get a form of contract from the home being considered before entering into any agreement. The people running this type of home will almost certainly be highly trained and professional carers and the home should have an in-house training scheme in operation for staff training purposes.

Selecting the right residential home for you

At first, the thought of selecting a home may seem a daunting task, but with an objective approach it need not be so. The first major hurdle has been crossed – your acceptance that you need residential care. Next you need to determine what type of home you want to live in.

One of the first things to decide is how you will pay to stay in the home. Will it be from your own resources, or will you need assistance? The next point to consider is the level of care you need. Are you fairly independent and active, or do you require a high level of support and supervision? Once you have established these two factors, the way forward is relatively easy.

Self-funding

If you are able to pay for a place in a home, this gives you a great deal of independence of choice, mainly because you will not need a local authority assessment of your care needs. Therefore, you can venture into the open market and make your own choice.

Securing a list of homes in your area or the immediate vicinity could not be simpler. The Registration and Inspection Unit of your local authority will have a list of all the homes in its catchment area and on its register, and they will supply you with this information. Other organisations have lists of residential homes which are likely to be categorised according to the type and level of care offered. Some of these organisations are listed below:

- Association of Approved Registered Care Homes
- British Federation of Care Home Proprietors
- Caresearch
- Counsel and Care for the Elderly
- Grace
- Help the Aged
- National Bed Line
- National Care Homes Association

It is advisable at this point to take stock of your financial situation and to determine how long you could sustain the residential home fees. Do keep in mind that fees are likely to increase. It is worth remembering that once your savings and capital fall to £8,000 or less, you will qualify for assistance with the payment of your fees. If you feel that you are likely to reach this figure sooner rather than later, it might be to your advantage to ask for an assessment of your care needs from the local authority. By doing this and alerting the authorities to a probable need for financial help in the foreseeable future, you will be setting up a care package that will be sustainable. However, should you leave the assessment until the time when you actually require financial help, you may find that the local authority will not enter into a contract with your existing home, and you may be forced to move. This could prove to be quite traumatic. If you think such a situation is likely to occur, you can get up-to-date information from your local Age Concern office or the Citizens' Advice Bureau.

Assisted funding

Assisted funding is available to those people whose savings and capital are £8,000 or less. Since April 1993 local authorities have been responsible for arranging and paying for residential care for those who need financial help. If you wish to enter residential care and require financial assistance to do so, you must apply to the Social Services Department of your local authority. They *must* then assess your need for care and arrange for a 'care package' to respond to these needs (see Chapter 1, 'The assessment process'). You should then be offered a place in a residential home which might be run by the local authority, a voluntary organisation, or privately. It is almost certain to be with an establishment with whom the council already has a contract. You may feel pressurised into accepting the place offered, but do remember that you have a *right of choice*, known as your 'preferred accommodation'. This right is safeguarded by law as long as the following conditions apply.

- The accommodation is suitable for your assessed needs.

- The person in charge of the home is prepared to provide the level of care under the local authority's usual conditions.
- The accommodation costs no more than the local authority would otherwise expect to pay.

If your chosen accommodation is suitable but not immediately available, the local authority should find you a temporary placement until the place of your choice is available.

Should the home of your choice cost more than the local authority would normally pay, it is still possible for you to take up residency provided a third party, usually a relative or charity, will make up the shortfall. You should exercise caution here, however, because there is no guarantee that any future increase in fees will be met equally by the parties involved. It is advisable to check with the local authority what system they intend to employ to cover situations like this, and then to set up a regular review procedure with the third party and the authority.

Other points to bear in mind are:

- A local authority *cannot* expect a third party (a relative or friend or a charity) to contribute towards fees if the home costs no more than the authority would usually expect to pay.
- The only person, apart from yourself, who can be expected to contribute towards the fees is your spouse or partner.
- Should the local authority want your spouse or partner to make a contribution towards the fees, it must go through the courts who will set an amount considered 'reasonable'.
- You should not be asked to pay extra if there is no available place at the authority's 'usual price'.

- If a local authority is unable to make an arrangement for a place in a suitable home at what it deems to be the usual price, it is the authority rather than the resident or a third party that must pay the extra cost.

Some guidelines

Before you set about the task of choosing the right home, it might be worthwhile to pause and give thought to what *you* expect from a residential care home. Making a list of these expectations could be extremely helpful when assessing what a home is actually offering you. The following list of expectations may be useful:

- To have a contract of residence, a brochure and statement of terms and conditions of residency, prior to admission;
- To receive a quality of service of a consistent standard that is appropriate and responsive to individual needs;
- To have your care evaluated and discussed at regular intervals with the management of the home and to be given genuine and informed choices of the options available for your future care;
- To be provided with homely, safe and clean accommodation of a high standard and encouraged to bring personal possessions into the home;
- To be given a choice of high quality, appetising and nourishing food appropriate to individual dietary needs and personal wishes;
- To be cared for by appropriately trained and qualified staff;
- To receive personal information on your condition and prospects, and to be informed of the person ultimately responsible for your care;
- To be able to retain the doctor of your choice whenever possible;

- To be allowed the chance to handle your own medicines when it is appropriate so to do;
- To receive medical and nursing care in a private place;
- To be encouraged and assisted in maintaining a high quality of life, with respect for individuality;
- To bathe, wash and use toilet facilities in private, or with assistance if you wish;
- To be allowed to maintain independence – choosing, whenever possible, your own level of freedom and lifestyle;
- To be persuaded to fulfil your human, emotional and social needs;
- To have your interests dealt with confidentially and your privacy respected;
- To have the right to follow the religion of your choice and fulfil your spiritual needs;
- To be safeguarded from discrimination on any grounds;
- To be addressed in a polite and proper manner;
- To be able to continue old friendships and encouraged to form new ones;
- To be able to receive visitors at any reasonable time;
- To have access to a telephone that is placed in a position of privacy;
- To participate in recreational activities and to be given the opportunity to develop new hobbies and pastimes;
- To be encouraged to use the facilities available to other people living in the community and assisted to make this possible;
- To have the right to consult a solicitor, adviser or advocate privately and have the right to be represented, when necessary, to put forward your own point of view;
- To be able to comment freely, or complain about, any aspect of the service provided by the home through

formal, or informal, channels; knowing that your views will be listened to and, wherever possible, accommodated.

Visiting and choosing a home

The problems in choosing the right home for yourself might be exacerbated by an apparent lack of vacancies, which could result in your feeling pressured into accepting the first opportunity that comes along. To prevent this situation from occurring it is advisable to give some thought to the sort of home you are looking for. This will make the selection task simpler and target your efforts in a more concentrated area. So what are you looking for?

Do you want a home with a small number of residents or a large complex catering for many people? Homes which cater for fewer than eight residents are not required to give 24-hour 'waking' care; perhaps a home like this would suit your need for independence. Or you may want the 'buzz' that a larger number of residents would bring to a home, with much happening and more coming and going. Once you have decided on the size of the home needed, you can start to cull your list; and armed with this shortlist you are then able to assess the viability of these homes. Before visiting homes, you might conduct a further process of elimination by telephoning the names on the list and by careful questioning cross off those that are of no interest. From those that remain you should then be in a position to put them into some order of preference.

Further considerations ought to be taken account of, however, and some of these might be:

* How far is the home from your present neighbour-hood?

- Is the area well served by public transport?
- Is there a bus stop or station close to the home?
- Is the home on a busy road; will there be traffic noise to contend with?
- Is the home affected by traffic pollution?
- Are there main roads to cross to reach local amenities?
- Do the staff encourage visits by family and friends?

You will probably have other aspects to consider, but the above suggestions should stimulate your thought process.

It might be advisable to visit the area a home is in to get a feel for the locality. Not only must you feel safe and happy in the home environment, but you should also find the surroundings comforting.

Once you have a final list, you should set up appointments for a visit and, if possible, ask a relative or friend to accompany you. On arrival at the home take some time to appraise the building's exterior. Does it look well maintained? Is the front garden well kept? Is the path to the house evenly paved and free from weeds and the like? (Moss is very slippery when wet.) Are there steps up to the front door, and how many? Is the surrounding neighbourhood of pleasing appearance?

When you meet the people who run the home, you will be under some pressure. They are likely to be very business-like and probably have a limited amount of time to spare you. On the other hand, you are likely to be feeling rather emotional. So when you enter the house, take your time, do not let anyone rush you. Remember that your first impressions, and perhaps your instincts, will alert you to possible problems. Trust your instincts. If your first reaction is one of discomfort, your feelings are more than likely correct. Should this happen, your questions and assessment should be critical in the extreme. There is probably a reason for your instinctive reaction, so find that reason.

If, however, your instinct and impressions are favourable, your assessment can be more positive and you can take on board your immediate reactions. Does the house seem warm and welcoming? Is it well furnished and are the curtains and carpets in good order? Are there any peculiar smells lingering around the house? Are the staff polite and friendly, and do the residents look well cared for? Are they engaged in any activities or just sitting around? Do they look clean and tidy, and do they seem alert?

All these factors give clear indications of how a home is run and should form the major part of your first impressions. It is also a good idea to spend some time talking to the staff and residents. You can learn a lot from the way they answer your questions, and their tone of voice.

What does the home offer?

It makes sense to visit a prospective home armed with a list of questions that you want answering. It is advisable not to try to commit the questions to memory but to have a written list which you refer to quite openly.

Here is a list of questions you might care to use.

- Does the home publish a brochure outlining the care and all the facilities it provides?
- What are the charges and what do these cover?
- Are there extra charges and if so what are they specifically?
- Is there a trial period for new entrants?
- Does the home encourage its residents to be independent, and where possible to do what they can for themselves?

- Can residents have a say in what they do in their daily lives?
- Is there a residents' committee?
- Are residents allowed to bring personal possessions with them, and if so, what is the range?
- Do residents have to share a room?
- If the accommodation is shared, does the resident have a say in whom they share with?
- Do rooms have their own en-suite facilities?
- Are there adequate and fully equipped lavatory facilities on each floor?
- Are special diets catered for?
- Is there a choice of menu each day?
- Can relatives and friends visit at any time, and are there private facilities for visits if necessary?
- Are there leisure activities; how are they arranged and is there usually a charge?
- Is there more than one common room – a place for reading and writing letters as well as for television?
- Does a mobile library visit the home, and is there provision for receiving newspapers and magazines?
- Can active residents visit the local shops or go out for walks?
- Is medication supervised?
- Can residents keep their own doctor or must they change to one more local?
- Are there adequate stair-lifts, lifts and fire escapes?
- Does the home accept people who are confused?
- What arrangements are made for hospital stays or short holidays – will a resident's bed be kept, and if so, at what cost?
- What arrangements are made for funerals and for payment if a resident dies?
- Does the home accept residents funded by the local authority, and does the contract state this?

- For residents receiving local authority support, when do they receive their personal expense allowance?

These are just the basic questions that ought to be asked, and you may have several more to add to the list. Make a note of these, and be sure to ask all the questions and ensure that you receive answers that you understand.

Your checklist

Having established your list of expectations and made a list of questions to be asked about a prospective home, it is a good idea to have a checklist divided into specific areas so that you can make notes alongside each item. Remember, you will be in a strange environment, people will be showing you different things and talking to you at the same time, so it is very likely you will find it difficult to concentrate. Having such a list to hand will be extremely valuable and help you to remember all the questions you need to ask. A suggested format is set out below:

Finances

- What do the fees include?
- What are the 'extras', if any?
- Can you afford the fees on a long-term basis?
- If there is a 'top up' portion, can you or your family afford this on a long-term basis?
- How often are the home fees increased?
- Can you afford regular fee increases?
- Will you have to move if you cannot meet the increased fees?
- How much will you have to pay when temporarily absent from the home?

Contracts

- Is there a written contract?

- Do you fulfil the terms of admission?
- What are the circumstances in which you may be asked to leave?
- Who is responsible for finding you alternative accommodation?
- What is the term of notice required by either side in order to cancel the contract?

It is advisable to take some time to read the contract through carefully and to seek advice from your family, friends, solicitor or Citizens' Advice Bureau. Do not be pressured into signing the contract until you are certain that the home is what you want.

Location

- Where is the home situated? Is the road quiet? Is there traffic noise?
- Is it close to family, friends and neighbours?
- Is the home convenient for shops, public transport, the local park and your doctor?
- Are there busy roads to cross to reach these amenities?
- Are there any hills en route?

The accommodation

- Will you be able to manage the steps in and around the home?
- Is there easy access for walking frames or wheelchairs throughout?
- Are the toilets and bathrooms easily accessible?
- How many communal rooms are there for residents' use?
- Is the dining room separate from the sitting room?
- Is there a quiet room and are there smoking and non-smoking areas?

- Will you have to share a room and, if so, will there be enough privacy?
- Can you have furniture and personal possessions in your room?
- Do the rooms smell fresh and clean?

Organisation of the home

- Are the meal times flexible?
- Is the menu varied, and are special diets catered for?
- Are the times for getting up and going to bed flexible?
- Do the staff respect the residents' privacy and knock on doors before entering rooms?
- Do you feel there are enough members of staff?
- How many people are on duty at night?

Other facilities

- Is there a garden?
- Are there organised leisure activities?
- What services are provided in the way of hairdressing, chiropody, library and laundry?
- Will your religious needs be catered for?
- Can you receive visitors at any time, and can they be seen in private?
- Are you allowed to eat in your room if you wish?
- Are you allowed to prepare your own drinks and light snacks?

Final points

- Are you *sure* that the fees are affordable?
- Is there a waiting list?
- If your care needs should change, what is likely to happen?
- Who is responsible for the decision making in this respect?

- Do the other residents look happy, clean and well cared for?
- Did you speak to any of them?
- What was your impression of what they had to say?
- How does the home brochure compare with your impressions?
- Can you arrange for a trial period of a month or so to see if the home and you are suited?
- Do you feel the home can offer you the care you need, and do you think you will be happy living there?
- Only you can decide if the home is for you. What do your instincts tell you?

Summary

After you have seen all there is to see about a home and have asked all the right questions and understood the answers, you will need time to reflect and confer with the person who accompanied you. Do not be rushed into making any decisions, and do not commit yourself to anything. Take all the time necessary to evaluate what you have seen and heard. Give careful thought to the cost implications and be certain that you can manage the fees; or, if you will be receiving financial help to pay the fees, make sure that the help is adequate and all proper safeguards are in place. If there are elements you are unsure about speak to those running the home again. If necessary, arrange to visit the home once more to satisfy yourself that it is as you remember. Perhaps you might ask for a trial period to see how you would fit in.

Do take the time to consider all aspects most carefully. Remember, you are choosing your future home, and your choice must be the right one.

Finding a nursing home

Since April 1993 and the deeper involvement in community care by local authorities, the dividing line between what constitutes a residential care home and a nursing home has become somewhat fuzzy. Almost certainly you will come into contact with both kinds of home during your research into care options, so it would be beneficial to know something about nursing homes. The majority are run privately by individuals, partnerships or companies; some are run by voluntary organisations, and a diminishing number are in the hands of local authorities under the auspices of the District Health Authority (DHA).

By law all nursing homes must register with the local DHA and are subject to inspection at least twice a year. The registration certificate must be displayed in a prominent position in the home and will specify the maximum number of people for whom the home can care.

The main difference between a nursing home and a residential home is that the person in charge of a nursing home must be a registered medical practitioner or a qualified nurse. The home must also provide full 24-hour nursing care by qualified staff.

The process of finding a suitable nursing home is very similar to that used in finding a residential one. If you are self-funding, you can select your own home and arrange for the services you require; your GP will need to be involved with your decision and may recommend a home for you. Obtaining a list of nursing homes in your locality is relatively simple.

You might care to contact the following:

- The registration officer for nursing homes at the District Health Authority;
- Your local Social Services Department;
- The secretary at your local hospital.

Other agencies offering help with advice and information are mentioned elsewhere in this book.

If you are in need of financial assistance, you will have to be assessed by the local authority, as already outlined. The process is the same as for residential care, except that more departments within the local council, and elsewhere, will be consulted because a health problem is involved. Your rights under the DHS and Community Care Act 1990 are not diminished.

The funding of nursing-home care follows the same pattern as residential care. However, because of the need for extra qualified staff and more concerted care provision, nursing homes tend to cost more to run and charge higher fees. As a result, there appears to be a trend towards directing people away from nursing-home care into residential-home care. If this should happen, you need to stand your ground and insist that your right to proper care is observed. It is unlawful for a local authority not to supply a service that it has a duty to provide, by reason of lack of funds.

4. Financing the Care Options

Whatever care option you choose, there is going to be a cost element involved which will have to be met by someone. Your own financial situation will determine whether you will pay all the care costs or whether you will receive some form of assistance. However, it might be appropriate to give an indication as to what are the cost implications of the care options discussed in this book.

Staying in your own home

Care and Repair and Staying Put are agencies which offer advice and practical help to elderly home owners on the repair or improvement of their homes.

These schemes are likely to entail some modifications to your home which could include rewiring, restructuring and some building work. There is almost certain to be a requirement for plans to be drawn up and a 'specialist' employed to see that all work is carried out to specification. Although some of this work may qualify for grant funding, the implication is that you will have to meet all the costs. You may be able to get help with these costs from outside sources such as charities, but the main point to bear in mind is that you still retain ownership. Your home will have a residual value. Note that if you are applying for a grant, you should not start work on any repairs or improvements before the grant is agreed.

Elderly private tenants who are experiencing problems with their landlords can seek advice from the Citizens' Advice Bureau, or the renovation grants centre of their local council, a housing advice centre, or the national office of Care and Repair.

Various grants are available for repairs and improvements through local authorities. Some work will qualify for a *mandatory grant* while other work may qualify for a *discretionary grant*. The size of the grant you get will depend on your income. If you are in receipt of Income Support, Council Tax Benefit, or Housing Benefit and are a home owner, or a private or housing association tenant, and over the age of 60, you may qualify for a *minor works grant* of up to £1,080.

Disabled facilities grants can cover all, or part, of the cost of adaptations such as installing a downstairs toilet, and some types of work attract mandatory grants. In a situation such as this, the renovation grants section of the local authority has a duty to consult with the Social Services Department. An occupational therapist will normally visit to assess the need, and the size of any grant awarded is determined by the level of income of the person applying for the grant.

For further information or advice, contact the Royal Association for Disability and Rehabilitation (RADAR). The Department of the Environment publishes a free booklet, *House Renovation Grants*, available from local authority offices.

Having care in your home

In all probability you will have to use your own income to meet the cost of such things as a home help, meals on wheels, laundry services and the like. As much of the help

FINANCIAL

WHO'S GOING TO FOOT THE BILL ?

As a nation we are living longer and the state has already sent warnings that it cannot care for all of us. It has never before been more essential that you plan ahead for a long, happy and financially secure retirement.

Trafalgar Financial Consultants Limited is a firm of independent financial advisers who can help you establish a plan for all of your life. For an initial discussion telephone Celeste Boucher or David Mount on 0171 240 6626 or alternatively write to:-

Trafalgar Financial Consultants Ltd, FREE POST LON5074, London, WC2H 9EQ

Trafalgar Financial Consultants Ltd is a member of Countrywide independent Advisers Ltd, a PIA member

you will receive is likely to be provided by voluntary organisations, the payment you will be asked to make could be quite reasonable.

Buying sheltered housing

This is just the same as selling your home and taking on another one. You will be liable for all legal costs, yours and the vendor's, as well as removal, and other ancillary costs. Then of course there will be the management service charge to meet and your contribution to the 'sinking fund'. Here again your home will retain a residual value.

Sheltered accommodation

This type of option is usually available only through charities or other non-profit making concerns. Their usual practice is to charge only what people can afford.

Residential or nursing home care

The major cost factor is going to be the payment of fees which vary according to the facilities on offer and in which part of the country the home is located. Generally speaking, establishments in the south east and Greater London are more expensive than elsewhere, though some coastal town homes can also be costly.

Residential homes owned by local authorities have their fees governed by law and are based on actual costs. Voluntary organisations set their fees according to their rules and regulations, and in some cases these are a lot lower than the equivalent private accommodation. Privately owned home fees are set by the owners and invariably carry an element of cost plus mark-up that reflects their need to be profitable.

More and more local authorities are buying their residential care requirements on the open market, and it is obvious that their purchasing power is having an effect on fees. While this may seem to be a good thing, it can disguise the fact that some homes which have a mix of self-funding and local authority residents, probably have a two-tier fee structure.

The likely minimum fees charged by residential care homes (based on fees acceptable to local authorities) for 1993/94 were:

Greater London: £240 per week (£12,480 per annum)
Outside London: £215 per week (£11,180 per annum)

As one can see, residential care does not come cheap.

Self-funding

Absolute freedom of choice as to type of home, its size, location and classification is yours when you are self-funding. Your only concern is whether you meet the conditions of admission. Be aware, though, that you will be entering into a commercial contract. The proprietors will be offering you a service for which you will be paying; therefore, even if there is no written contract, in law one does exist.

The proprietors will want to assure themselves that you can meet the financial commitment and will inevitably ask you a number of searching questions and will take up credit references. They may also ask for a deposit, or an advance payment of several weeks' fees; or they may ask you to supply a guarantor, usually a family member. If after these investigations they refuse to accept you, you are entitled to ask the reason. It could be they have spotted a weakness in your financial situation and, if so, you ought to know what it entails. They do not have to give you a reason for their refusal; but quite often, if they are questioned properly, they will tell you.

It is very important for you to be certain that your weekly income can be maintained in the long term. It is not unusual for private residential care homes to have fees in excess of £300 per week for self-funding residents. This fact would mean that you would need to have an annual income of at least £15,600 after tax just to meet the fees, and of course you would need more than this to take account of personal expenses. When making this assessment of your income long term, remember that fees are more than likely to increase. Will your income rise at the same rate?

If you are unable to meet the cost of residential or nursing home care from your income and assets and the amount of these is less than £8,000, then you should claim Income Support and financial help from the local authority, as explained in detail on pages 82–89.

Maximising your income

In determining how you can manage the cost of care, you will need to make a complete appraisal of your finances. Perhaps with the help of your family, close friends or an independent financial adviser, you could consider the following factors:

- Should you sell your home and invest the proceeds to increase your income in the future?
- Do you wish to retain your home to 'pass on' when you die?
- Can you raise money from your home without necessitating its sale?
- Do you need to switch investments from 'growth' to 'income'?
- Are you receiving your full entitlement to the State Retirement Pension as well as other benefits?
- Do you qualify for any other benefit such as Attendance Allowance, owing to your physical condition?
- If you opt for residential or nursing home care what is the amount of the top-up element – the difference between the fee charged by the home and your weekly income, including Retirement Pension, your occupational pension, Attendance Allowance, etc? Is the gap between the two elements likely to grow?

There are various other factors that can be explored and require evaluating. For example, if you decide to remain in your own home, you may be able to use its value as capital.

Money from the value of your home

There are several financial schemes available which allow you to receive capital or income against the equity in your home; and it is important to remember that, except for home reversion plans (see page 78), these are all credit schemes of one form or another. It is essential that you check all details of any offer very carefully, and it is highly recommended that you seek expert advice.

A number of companies active in this sector have formed the Safe Home Income Plan (SHIP) Campaign which sets out a strict code of practice. Key features of the code are a requirement that the company sets out the pros and cons of the schemes in a clear and adequate manner and that no deal should be finalised without the clearance of a client's solicitor.

SHIP Campaign
Hinton and Wild (Home Plans) Ltd
374 Ewell Road
Surbiton
Surrey
KT6 7BB
Tel: 0181 390 8166

Home income plans

One way to raise income against the equity in your home is through a home income plan. Usually, an interest-only loan is made against a proportion of the value of your home, but you retain full ownership of the property.

The loan is used to buy an annuity from an insurance company which provides income for life; however, part of the income will have to go towards paying the interest on the loan. The loan itself is repaid in full when the property is sold.

Before proceeding with a home income plan, you should look into all aspects of the transaction and take professional advice from your solicitor and an independent financial adviser.

The following list suggests what features you ought to be aware of:

- Interest rates may vary and over the long term are likely to increase. Remember that the interest will have to be paid out of your income.
- Be certain what the interest-rate factor is and how it will be applied.
- When the loan is finally repaid it will reduce the amount available to your beneficiaries.
- If you are in receipt of Income Support or other means-tested benefits, the amount of annuity received will be regarded as income, and the amount of benefit will be reduced accordingly.
- There are likely to be costs involved in buying a home income plan by way of arrangement, survey and legal fees.
- There are several drawbacks to annuities, not the least of which is the poor return if the holder or holders die early.
- There is a minimum age both for individuals and couples (cumulative) wanting to invest in one of these plans.

The following commercial enterprises offer home income plans. It is strongly recommended that you get professional advice before entering into any agreement.

Allchurches Life Assurance Ltd
Carlyle Life Assurance Company Ltd
Hinton and Wild (Home Plans) Ltd

Home reversion schemes

With these schemes you sell your home to the reversion company but you and your partner then have the right to live in the home for life as legally protected tenants, usually rent free.

You receive a proportion of the value of your home outright, usually not more than 50 per cent but generally less, and dependent upon your life expectancy. In some schemes it is possible to sell off a part of the property. The amount realised can be paid to you as a lump sum or in the form of an annuity.

Some other points worth considering about reversion schemes:

- Your beneficiaries will not inherit your home.
- It is unlikely that a reversion company would be interested in acquiring a leasehold property.
- You are likely to remain responsible for all repairs and maintenance.
- You may be restricted if the need to move house arises.
- There is likely to be a hefty arrangement fee, usually between 1 and 2 per cent of the value of the property.
- If you are in receipt of a means-tested state benefit, the lump sum or extra income could result in your losing part, or all, of your entitlement.

Here is a list of financial institutions offering home reversion schemes:

Brent Reversions Services Ltd
Carlyle Life Assurance Company Ltd
Cavendish Home Reversions Ltd
Hinton and Wild (Home Plans) Ltd
Home and Capital Trust Ltd
Investment Property Reversions Ltd
Regentsmead Group
Residential Home Reversions Ltd
Sovereign Reversions plc
Stalwart Assurance Company Ltd

Annuities

Purchasing an annuity involves paying a lump sum to an

insurance company which then pays you an income for life. The amount of income you receive depends largely on the capital sum you provided but more importantly on your life expectancy and the interest rates prevailing when you bought the annuity.

There are various schemes available, and it is advisable to shop around, but the fundamental criterion as to how well you do will be the insurance company's assessment of your life expectancy.

With an annuity, tax is usually deducted at source, and if you are not liable to tax it must be reclaimed from the Inland Revenue office that holds your file. It is possible to have a 'capital protected' annuity which, while paying slightly less income, will return some of the capital in the event of your dying within five years.

It is worth noting that companies providing annuities are registered with Lautro Ltd (LAUTRO). However, this organisation will cease to exist after October 1995 and will be incorporated within the Personal Investment Authority. Companies already registered with LAUTRO are not necessarily required to register with PIA but they are required to register with a 'regulatory body'. Companies who provide lump sum payments are not required to register.

Check your income tax liability

Any calculations made or conclusions reached regarding the cost of care should take into account any income tax liability that exists, and an appraisal of your tax situation is imperative. As a general rule, older people are liable to pay income tax if their gross taxable income exceeds the amount of their tax allowance.

Investment income is classed as taxable income, except for TESSAs, Premium Bond winnings and National

Savings Certificates. Interest on bank or building society accounts is usually taxed at source. If, however, your gross income, which includes interest income, does not exceed the amount of your tax allowances, you can ask the bank or building society to pay the gross interest. In order to do this, you will need to complete form R85, obtainable from banks, building societies, post offices and tax offices. Further information concerning relief from tax or the refund of tax already paid is available in Inland Revenue leaflets IR11 and IR112.

Retirement pensions and occupational pensions usually count as taxable income (see Inland Revenue Leaflet IR4 *Income Tax and Pensioners*).

State benefits may also count as taxable income, and as a guide, the following list is currently applicable:

Taxable benefits

- Retirement pensions, including any invalidity addition;
- Widow's Pension, Widow's Allowance and Widowed Mother's Allowance;
- Invalid Care Allowance;
- Industrial death benefit (if paid as a pension);
- Statutory Sick Pay.

Non-taxable benefits

- Sickness Benefit;
- Invalidity Benefit, including Invalidity Allowance;
- Severe Disablement Allowance;
- Industrial Injuries Disablement Benefit;
- Disability Living Allowance;
- Disability Working Allowance;
- Housing Benefit and Council Tax Benefit;
- Income Support for people aged 60 or more (and those

who receive this benefit without having to be available for work);

- Christmas Bonus for pensioners;
- Attendance Allowance;
- Disablement pensions from the armed forces, police, fire brigade, merchant navy;
- Additions for dependent children;
- War Widow's Pension and allowances;
- Social Fund payments.

The personal tax allowances are higher for people aged 65 to 74 and higher still for those aged 75 or more. However, these higher allowances are reduced if your total gross income exceeds a specified amount (see Inland Revenue Leaflet IR4A *Income Tax Age Allowance*).

Assistance and information on any income tax-related matter can be obtained from your local PAYE Enquiry Office (the address and telephone number can be found in the telephone directory).

To repeat, before entering into any agreement for residential care be sure the fees are within your capabilities, and that any arrangement for outside assistance to meet the top-up element is securely in place.

Assisted funding for residential and nursing home care

If you have savings and capital of £8,000 or less, you should qualify for financial support in respect of care fees. It is the responsibility of your local authority to provide that support if they think there is a duty for them to do so.

If you entered a registered residential home before 1 April 1993 you will have what are known as 'preserved rights'. However, if you were in a 'small home' – that is, one with fewer than four residents – prior to April 1993, you will not have these preserved rights.

Financially supported entry into a registered private or voluntary residential home is now controlled by the local authority which makes placements in suitable homes in the light of care assessments. If a need for residential care is agreed, the local authority will find a place in a suitable home, enter into a legal contract with that home, and take the legal responsibility for paying the fees.

As a result of the changes the whole aspect of assisted funding is rather convoluted and has become somewhat complicated. It is important that you become conversant with the various aspects of assisted funding, but in doing so you will see certain elements of duplication. This is because the Benefits Agency (DSS), who were the sole providers of financial support, now work in tandem with local authorities who are now the main providers of such assistance. Although local authorities generally follow the line that the Benefits Agency took, there is no legal requirement of them to do so, and as a result some of their provision may differ in various ways. The following is an explanation of the different areas of assisted funding.

Preserved rights to Income Support

If you entered a registered residential care home, having four or more residents, before 1 April 1993 and were paying fees from your own resources you have 'preserved rights' to Income Support at the higher level once your savings and capital are reduced to £8,000 or less.

If you need to make a claim in this respect, complete form SP1 (available from the Benefits Agency) or write a letter which should contain your name, the name and address of the home and the date of your admission (you will still be required to complete form SP1).

Maximum levels of income support towards residential care home fees (rates in force until April 1996)

Category of care	Greater London £	Outside Greater London £
Homes for the elderly	231	197
Homes for the elderly in receipt of higher rate Attendance Allowance, or Disability Living Allowance (higher care component); or who are registered blind	261	227
Registered home for the mentally ill	241	207
Registered home for those dependent on drugs or alcohol	241	207
Registered home for mentally handicapped people	271	237
Registered homes for the physically disabled where: (a) the claimant was registered disabled before pension age or able to prove disability before pension age	301	267
(b) disability arose after pension age	231	197
Other categories	231	197

In addition to the above rates, a claimant will be paid an allowance for personal expenses (currently £13.35 per week).

Maximum levels of income support towards nursing home fees (rates in force until April 1996)

Category of care	Greater London £	Outside Greater London £
Nursing homes for the elderly	334	295
Nursing homes for the mentally ill	335	296
Nursing homes for those dependent on drugs or alcohol	335	296
Nursing homes for the mentally handicapped	340	301
Nursing homes for the terminally ill	334	295
Nursing homes for the physically disabled where: (a) claimant was registered disabled before pension age or able to prove disability before pension age	370	331
(b) disability arose after pension age	334	295
Other categories	334	295

A nursing home does not need to be registered to supply a specific category of care. The Income Support limit applies to the type of care that is provided. The claimant will receive an allowance for personal expenses (currently £13.35 per week).

All documents *must* be signed by you or your recognised appointee and be forwarded to the Benefits Agency office that covers the area where the home is situated. Income Support can only be backdated under very special circumstances, so do not delay in making your claim.

The amount of Income Support you receive will depend on the type of care you require and will have established maximum limits, which are usually upgraded annually. There are separate limits for residential care and nursing home care. The following tables show the amounts of Income Support allowable toward fees within and outside the Greater London area.

It is worth checking with the local Benefits Agency office if a particular home falls within the Greater London area. Some parts of Essex, Hertfordshire and Surrey are counted as being part of Greater London even though they are outside the official boundary.

Claiming Income Support

Income Support is a means-tested benefit and is contingent upon the claimant meeting strict criteria. It is available to people whose *total* income falls below amounts prescribed by law.

For people over the age of 60, the general criteria are:

- They must reside in the United Kingdom;
- They do not work more than 15 hours a week;
- They do not have a partner who works more than 15 hours a week;
- They do not have savings and capital (including a partner's savings and capital) over £8,000.

If both partners in a couple qualify for Income Support either one of them can claim it.

The benefit paid is the difference between an amount prescribed by law (the 'applicable amount') and any income you have from other sources, less any 'disregards'. For people living in residential care homes or nursing homes, there are special rules for calculating Income Support.

The applicable amount is made up of prescribed personal allowances, additions for dependent children, extra entitlements due to pensioners, carers and disabled people, payments for mortgage interest and certain other housing costs not usually covered by Housing Benefit.

When calculating income your savings and capital up to £3,000 are disregarded; thereafter, up to a limit of £8,000, each £250 or part of £250 is treated as income of £1 per week. There is no entitlement to benefit if your savings and capital, or your partner's savings and capital, or your joint savings and capital, exceed £8,000.

If you qualify for Income Support you should be able to claim it if you go to live in a voluntary or private care home and are required to meet the fees yourself.

However, the Benefits Agency will put a ceiling on the amount of fees to be taken into consideration. This limit is based upon the category of care that the home is registered with the local authority to provide, but if the care home is registered in more than one category the limit is set according to the level of care being provided for you.

What you receive is the prescribed maximum amount, or the actual fee charged by the home if this is the lower, minus your income. It is important to remember that Attendance Allowance, Constant Attendance Allowance, and the personal care content of Disability Living Allowance are all treated as income.

If you are entering a residential care or nursing home on a permanent basis, any property that you own, or partially own, will be taken into consideration when determining your entitlement to Income Support. Property includes the home you own and if its value exceeds £8,000, you will not receive Income Support unless and so long as the property remains occupied either wholly or in part by your spouse, cohabitee, or a relative who is over 60 or who is incapacitated.

Should you decide to sell the property, its value may be disregarded for up to six months, sometimes longer while the sale goes through. If, during this period, your savings are reduced to less than £8,000, you can claim Income Support.

Your spouse's income and capital will not be taken into account unless your admission to a home is temporary, or you are both admitted together, but if a spouse is able to contribute towards the fees charged by a residential or nursing home, it is likely to be taken into consideration when your Income Support assessment is made.

Where the fees charged by the care home exceed the prescribed maximum, any payment you receive towards the balance, from whatever source is *not* regarded as income.

Finally, should you experience difficulty in securing care at the levels of benefit mentioned above, it is suggested that you advise your Member of Parliament of your predicament and ask him or her to refer the matter to the Secretary of State for Social Security.

For further information, see DSS leaflet IS20 'A Guide to Income Support'.

Claiming Attendance Allowance and Disability Living Allowance

You are entitled to claim these benefits provided you fulfil the qualifying conditions.

Attendance Allowance is payable to people over the age of 65 who have either a physical or sensory disability, or both, and who need help with personal care or supervision. As an example you should qualify if you need help in getting dressed, washing, going to the toilet or making a hot meal regularly. There are two levels at which Attendance Allowance can be paid: a lower rate for people who need personal care or attention during the day *or* at night, and a higher rate for those who need personal care or attention during the day *and* at night.

Usually you have to meet the criteria for six months before benefit is actually paid, but there are special rules for people who are terminally ill.

The benefit is *not means tested* and it is not affected by your income or savings. However, it is important to bear in mind that DLA is treated as income entitlement when assessing your entitlement to benefits other than Attendance Allowance.

If you live alone or with someone else, you should claim Attendance Allowance; what matters is the fact that you *need care and attention*. For further information ask for leaflet DS702 or claim pack DS2 from your local Benefits Agency (Social Security Office) or telephone Benefits Enquiry Line on Freephone 0800 882 200.

People who become disabled before reaching the age of 65 should claim the *Disability Living Allowance* (DLA) provided they meet the following conditions:

- They need help with personal care, supervision or to have someone watching over them; or

- They are unable to walk or have great difficulty walking, or need to be accompanied when walking outdoors; or
- They need help with both of these.

The DLA does not depend on National Insurance contributions, is not means tested and will not normally affect other benefits or pensions received. The care component of DLA, however, is normally counted as income where a person is receiving Income Support in a registered care home. DLA has two parts: a 'care component', paid at one of three levels, and a 'mobility component' which has two different levels. To qualify for DLA you must meet one or more of the care or mobility conditions as set out below:

- You must be under 65 years of age or become disabled before your 65th birthday and not yet have reached 66. If you do not meet this criterion you should claim Attendance Allowance.
- You should also have fulfilled the day and/or night conditions (see below) for at least three months and expect to continue to do so for the following six months. However, there are special rules for people who are terminally ill.
- You must normally reside in the United Kingdom when you make a claim and have been here for at least 26 weeks during the last 12 months. This does not necessarily apply to those claiming under the special rules for the terminally ill.

Day conditions. You will fulfil this condition if you are so disabled that you need frequent help throughout the day with normal daily routines such as eating and drinking, getting up and down stairs, washing and going to the toilet. You also qualify if you require continual supervision throughout the day to prevent you substantially endangering yourself or others.

Night conditions. You will fulfil this condition if you are so disabled that you need prolonged periods (of at least 20 minutes' duration) or repeated (at least twice a night) periods of attention to help you in and out of bed and to go to the toilet. You will also qualify if someone else needs to stay awake for prolonged periods or frequent intervals throughout the night to ensure that you do not substantially endanger yourself or others.

Finding the top-up element

If you find that because of your individual situation there is a top-up of fees to be arranged and you have no family to turn to for this, you might like to consider the following:

The Association of Charity Officers will supply you with a list of their members which may suggest which organisations to approach.

Other organisations for you to consider are Counsel and Care for the Elderly, Help the Aged and Age Concern England.

Various funding examples

The following examples show how you can get help with the fees for residential and nursing home care.

Assistance from charities

There is a number of charitable organisations that can be approached for help with the cost of care if you are in need, but most of them will expect you to have tried all possible statutory avenues and family resources first. It is likely that support for your application from a social worker or your doctor would be most helpful and, in fact, most societies insist upon a professional assessment accompanying the application.

You will need to determine which charity best suits your requirements. Some societies consider one-off grants only, others are only concerned with continuing support, such as helping to meet top-up costs for residential and nursing home care.

Example A

An elderly person having savings and capital totalling £2,500 lives in a registered residential care home where the weekly fees are £197.00

	£	£
Income Support allowance towards fees		197.00
Personal expenses allowance		13.35
Claimant's maximum assessed need		210.35
Less personal income		
State Retirement Pension	58.85	
Attendance Allowance	31.20	90.05
Amount of Income Support payable (assessed need less personal income)		120.30
Outcome		
Weekly fee	197.00	
Total income inclusive of personal allowance	**210.35**	

Claimant's income and Income Support entitlement exactly meet the fees charged by the home.

Example B

This elderly person has been paying the fees out of his or her own resources but savings and capital have been reduced to £7,000. The person is also in receipt of the higher rate of Attendance Allowance. The home is in Greater London, and the weekly fees are £280.

	£	£
Income Support allowance towards fees		261.00
Personal expenses allowance		13.35
Claimant's maximum assessed need		**274.35**
Less personal income (Assumed income from capital of £7,000 is £16.00):		
State Retirement Pension	58.85	
Higher Attendance Allowance	46.70	
Income from capital	16.00	121.55
Amount of Income Support payable (assessed need less personal income)		152.80
Outcome		
Weekly fees	280.00	
Total income (inclusive of personal allowance)	**274.35**	

The claimant's income plus the Income Support entitlement, *excluding* the personal allowance element, gives a shortfall of £19.00 per week.

Example C

This person lives in a nursing home in Greater London where the fees are £390 per week. She/he has capital and savings of £6,000 and joint ownership of a house occupied by a spouse.

	£	£
Income Support allowance towards fees		334.00
Personal expenses allowance		13.35
Claimant's maximum assessed need		347.35
Less personal income (house fully disregarded; assumed income from capital of £6,000 is £12.00):		
State Retirement Pension	58.85	
Higher Attendance Allowance	46.70	
Income from capital	12.00	117.55
Amount of Income Support: (assessed need less personal income)		229.80
Outcome		
Weekly fees	390.00	
Total income (inclusive of personal allowance)	**347.35**	

The shortfall, not including personal expenses, is £42.65 per week.

It might be more beneficial to your case to look for a charity with which you can claim a connection – perhaps a local trust for which your qualification may be many years of residence in the area. There are likely to be local branches of the Round Table, Rotary, Lions, Foresters or

Buffaloes. You may have an association with a bene-volent society through previous employment or trade union affiliation; perhaps you have connections either personally or through your family with an ex-service organisation.

Professional people might seek advice and information from such organisations as Homelife; Distressed Gentlefolk's Aid Association; Friends of the Elderly and Gentlefolk's Help; Guild of Aid for Gentlepeople; or the Royal United Kingdom Beneficent Association.

Funding special situations

Hospitalisation
If you have to go into hospital while you are in a residential home, you can retain your preserved right (see page 83) to get Income Support for up to 52 weeks. If the home charges you for your room while you are in hospital, you will receive Income Support towards the fees for the first six weeks. Thereafter the Benefits Agency will pay a higher hospital personal allowance and a retaining fee which is either 80 per cent of your Income Support or the actual retaining fee levied by the home, whichever is the smaller. If your stay in hospital exceeds 52 weeks, you will lose your preserved right to Income Support and will need to be assessed by the local authority prior to your discharge.

Holidays or extended leave
You can be away from the home for a period not exceeding 13 weeks; and retain your preserved right (see page 83), and if the home charges you for your room, the Benefits Agency (DSS) will pay a retaining fee for up to four weeks. The level of retaining fee will be at 80 per cent of your Income Support or the fee the home actually charges, whichever is the smaller. In addition you may also claim Income Support at the normal levels for the

period you are away from the home as long as you do not leave the country. After 13 weeks' absence, you will forfeit your preserved rights and will need local authority assessment on your return.

Alternative accommodation

You may have to move to another home if you have been living in a registered care home for at least 12 months and paying your own way, but your savings and capital are now reduced to £8,000 or less and you can no longer afford the fees. The Benefits Agency will pay the full fee for up to 13 weeks to allow sufficient time for you to find alternative accommodation.

Funding arrangements since April 1993

People who have entered a registered private or voluntary care home since 1 April 1993 no longer qualify for the higher rate of Income Support, which included a contribution towards the care costs in the home. Now that it is a local authority's responsibility to pay for these care costs, you will only qualify for the normal levels of Income Support. In other words, your financial status is means tested twice – once by the Benefits Agency and again by the local authority.

If you are eligible for Income Support and moving into a registered private or voluntary care home you will receive the following:

- Basic rate of Income Support; plus
- Any premiums you are entitled to; and a
- Residential allowance.

These elements will be taken into account by the Social Services Department when it calculates your contribution towards the fees. Payments for fees will usually be made up from the following elements:

- *Personal income* (retirement pension, occupational pension, income from savings)
- *Income Support* (personal allowance, premiums, residential allowance)
- *Local authority contribution* (the difference between personal income plus Income Support – (if payable) – and the approved fee).

A person who enters a registered care home and has savings and capital of £8,000 or less is expected to contribute all their weekly income, less a personal allowance element of £13.35, to the local authority. Thus, if your weekly income is £150 and the home's fees are £200, you will retain £13.35 and pay the balance, £136.65, to the local authority. You should never pay *more* than the actual fees to the council and should never be left with less than £13.35 per week for personal expenditure.

The Benefits Agency will calculate the basic Income Support element in the following way (based on the rates in force until 6 April 1995).

The 'applicable amount' currently varies between £65.10 (people 65 years to 74 years) and £71.65 (people over 74 years) plus a residential allowance of £51.00 a week (£57.00 a week for Greater London). Therefore the following applies:

Income Support element

	65 to 74 years £	over 74 years £
Applicable amount	65.10	71.65
Residential allowance	51.00	51.00
	116.10	122.65

Thus your income, if necessary, will be topped up to these amounts. However, if your savings and capital are between £3,000 and £8,000, you must deduct £1.00 for every £250 or part thereof, in respect of the difference. So, for example, if you have £4,900 of savings, the amounts shown above would be reduced by £8.00.

Income disregards

Certain classes of income are disregarded which means they are ignored by both the Benefits Agency and the local authority. Other types of income are partially disregarded, and this means that £10.00 can be ignored but the balance will be taken into account. The following list is an *indication* of what a person over the age of 60 might expect to have disregarded or partially disregarded; it is not a definitive list.

Fully disregarded

- Mobility component of Disability Living Allowance
- Mobility Allowance
- Mobility Supplement
- Special War Widow's Pension (payments made to a widow whose spouse died from injuries or illness attributed to service which terminated before 31 March 1973)
- Gallantry Awards (Victoria Cross, George Cross, or equivalent made by another country)
- Pensioners' Christmas Bonus
- Charitable payments which are intended and used to pay for a specific item not covered by the home's fees, such as a television set.

Partially disregarded

- War Disablement Pension

- Civilian War Injury Pension
- War Widow's Pension
- Civil List Pensions (awarded by the Queen for distinguished service to the nation).

Even if you have several payments that attract the £10.00 disregard, only one £10 disregard can be allowed. However, you can have a fully disregarded payment and a partially disregarded payment.

Definitions of capital

Capital includes savings, National Savings certificates and accounts, income bonds, stocks and shares, premium bonds and property (including your own home).

Benefits Agency (DSS) definitions

Property

- The value of property owned by the claimant is usually treated as capital to be used towards fees, until the total capital is reduced to £8,000.
- The value of property being sold by the claimant, and being used towards fees, can be disregarded as a capital asset for six months (sometimes longer) while the sale is completed. If the claimant's other capital assets are below £8,000, Income Support can be claimed during this period.
- Property occupied by a spouse will be ignored as capital.
- Where ownership of a property is shared with anyone other than your partner, the value of the property will be divided equally for Income Support purposes.
- If a property is owned by two people in unequal proportions, ownership will be classed as 50 per cent each. However, this may differ under certain circum-

stances – if, for instance, there is a beneficial owner who is not the legal owner. A beneficial owner is a person with a beneficial interest, for example, a son or daughter who pays the mortgage or has paid for a share of the property but who, for whatever reasons, cannot be named as legal owner.

- A property occupied by an aged or incapacitated relative can be disregarded.

The following are defined as relatives: parents (including an adoptive parent), parents-in-law; a son or son-in-law; a daughter or daughter-in-law; a step-parent, step-son, step-daughter, a brother, sister, the spouse of any of these; grandparent or grandchild; uncle, aunt, nephew, niece.

Savings

- There is an assumed income of £1.00 each week for every £250, or part thereof, of capital in excess of £3,000 up to the limit of £8,000.
- If there are joint savings held in a joint account, they will be divided equally. The claimant entering care will be assessed on their half of the savings plus any held in their own name.
- Where the claimant and spouse have their own separate accounts, the claimant entering care will be assessed on his or her savings only.

Local authority definitions

Property

- The authority has the discretion to disregard a person's property where someone other than a relative (as detailed in the previous section) lives there.
- If a carer, who is not an aged or incapacitated relative, has been living in the person's home, the local

authority may disregard the property until it is no longer occupied or is sold.

- Any decision taken to disregard the property will mean that the local authority will incur higher costs in placing the person in a care home. This is because the Benefits Agency does not have to take the same view, so consequently the person entering care would not qualify for Income Support.
- Whereas the local authority can disregard a property, it can recoup its costs by putting a 'charge' against the property. This must be detailed in a contract between you and the local authority and means that any monies accruing from the date of admittance can be recovered when the property is eventually sold.
- Should the authority decide not to disregard a property, it can make an assessment of the value and then put a 'charge' on it and defer payment until a sale is arranged.

Savings

- A local authority views savings in exactly the same way as the Benefits Agency.

Example of local authority funding

The following example shows how the local authority system operates. (Sums used are based on rates in force until 5 April 1996.)

A person aged 79 and having savings of £4,900 enters a registered private residential care home in the Greater London area. The placement has been arranged by the local authority following an assessment of care needs. The home the person has chosen has fees that are higher than the authority will pay, but a third party has agreed to top up the difference of £22.50 per week.

	£	£
Fee for home (weekly)		212.50
Fee for local authority alternative		190.00
Third-party contributions		22.50

Income

	£	£
State Retirement Pension	58.85	
Assumed income (from capital of £4,900, this is £8.00)	8.00	66.85

Applicable amount

	£	£
Personal allowance	46.50	
Higher Pensioner premium	25.15	
Residential allowance	57.00	128.65

Income Support 61.80
(Applicable amount less
personal income)

Outcome

Resident's contribution towards home fees

Income	66.85
Less personal allowance (£13.35)	53.50
Income Support	61.80
Third-party contribution	22.50
Total contribution:	137.80

Local authority contribution

Fee for home	212.50
Resident's contribution (including third party)	137.80
Local authority contribution	74.70

Spouse's liability

Except in the case of a temporary admission to a care home, or the admission of both husband and wife, the income and capital of each partner must be assessed separately for the purpose of Income Support. However, local authorities always assess people separately even in the event of a temporary admission. A husband or wife may be classed as a *liable relative* and asked to contribute towards the maintenance of a spouse who is reliant on public funding. Unless the local authority or Benefits Agency obtains a court order, a payment is voluntary and should never be more than can realistically be afforded in the long term.

Should a spouse be deemed a liable relative, it is imperative that the level of their weekly contribution is discussed with their local authority or the *Liable Relatives Officer* at the Benefits Agency dealing with the claim, whichever is the most appropriate. It would also be advisable for the liable relative to seek legal advice.

Temporary absence

In the event of your being absent from the home because of hospitalisation you will receive your full applicable amount for a maximum of six weeks. Should you be absent for any other reason, such as holidays or a family visit, the residential allowance will be paid for up to three weeks only. This is only applicable when you intend to return to the same home. The local authority, however, has discretion to choose if they will continue to pay their contribution to your care costs. Because of this discretionary power it is advisable to ascertain the local authority's financial policy on temporary absences before making your initial arrangements for care.

5. Managing Your Financial Affairs

In today's complex world we seem to be bombarded with changes to most aspects of our daily lives, and nowhere is this more apparent than in the matter of personal finances. Banks and building societies operate electronic banking systems, direct debiting, a host of different savings and investment plans, they even sell insurance. Is it any wonder, therefore, that many people find the whole subject complicated and confusing?

We know that as we grow older we are less able to cope with change, and too much change can sap our self-confidence. If you feel that you need help in managing your financial affairs and the collection of benefits the following information may be of help.

Authorising others to act for you

Agency to collect social security benefits

If you have difficulty in visiting a post office to collect your benefits you may nominate someone to act as your 'agent' to collect the money, but not spend it, on your behalf. All that is required is for the declaration on the reverse of the pension order to be completed. Should the arrangement need to be long term an 'agency card' can be obtained from your local Benefits Agency.

Appointee to receive social security benefits

If a person who is entitled to social security benefits is unable to act for themselves, a representative of the Secretary of State for Social Security may, on receipt of a written application, appoint someone to make claims and to receive benefits, and to spend them, on the claimant's behalf. The person usually appointed will be a close relative or friend who lives with or frequently visits the claimant.

Third party mandate

This is usually used by people who are mentally capable but physically unable to visit a bank or building society and need someone to act on their behalf. It is necessary for you to contact the bank or building society to inform them of your needs and the completion of a form of authorisation is usually all that is required. Other institutions, however, require a separate form of authorisation for each transaction.

Power of attorney (ordinary) or enduring power of attorney

If you feel there is a need to appoint an attorney it is important that you understand the legal requirements and make the correct appointment. To help you decide which is more appropriate to your needs you should determine whether you want someone to act for you temporarily or under your supervision, in which case an ordinary power of attorney will suffice. If, however, you want someone to act for you now and if you should become mentally incapable in the future, or you wish someone to act for you *should* you become mentally incapable then an enduring power of attorney would be appropriate.

The person wishing to appoint an attorney is known as

the 'donor' while the person appointed is called a 'donee' or 'attorney'. A power of attorney provides a legal document which proves the powers of the 'donee' and the document may be purchased from a law stationer, such as Solicitors Law Stationery Society Ltd or Oyez Stationery Ltd. A solicitor will also draw up the form for you. It is important to remember that the ordinary power of attorney is only valid while the donor is capable of giving instructions. If the donor becomes mentally ill and no longer capable of supervising or directing the attorney then all powers of attorney cease immediately.

An enduring power of attorney (EPA) is a legal document appointing one or more persons to act for someone who feels that they may become incapable of managing their affairs at some time in the future. However, the document must be signed (executed) while the donor is capable of understanding the nature and effect of appointing an enduring power. An EPA must be in the form prescribed by the Enduring Powers of Attorney (Prescribed Form) Regulations 1990 and the form can be purchased from a law stationer or drawn up for the donor by a solicitor. It is important to note that the attorney should sign the document as soon as possible after the donor has signed and certainly before the donor becomes incapable of understanding the nature of the enduring power. Should the donor become incapable before the attorney has signed, the donor's 'intervening incapacity' automatically revokes the enduring power. In view of the complicated procedures as defined in the Enduring Powers of Attorney Act 1985 it is recommended that the advice of a solicitor is sought.

Court of Protection

If a person is unable to manage their financial affairs due to the deterioration of their mental state, and there is no enduring power of attorney in force, then application can be made to the Court of Protection on their behalf. The Court of Protection is an office of the Supreme Court and exists to protect and manage the financial affairs and property of people who are unable to manage for themselves due to mental disorder.

The Court can authorise two ways in which to administer the person's affairs:

1. The appointment of a receiver to manage the estate;
2. By a Short Procedure Order.

For the Court to exercise jurisdiction over a person it must be satisfied that 'in the light of the medical evidence the person is suffering from a mental disorder and is incapable, as a result of said disorder, of managing their financial affairs'. The person is then described as a patient.

The Court of Protection becomes involved only if something needs to be done to protect the patient's assets or to enable them to be used for the patient's benefit.

Information can be obtained from: Enquiries Branch, Court of Protection, Stewart House, 24 Kingsway, London WC2B 6JX. Tel: 0171 269 7300/7358.

Once again, it is advisable that advice and assistance be obtained from a solicitor in order that the interests of all parties are best served.

Making a will

Generally, we all accept that making a will is a good thing, and a large number of us are going to do it next week!

A will makes people aware of what we would like to happen when we die, who we want to benefit from our estate, and those we do not. People are left in no doubt as to our wishes, and as long as the will is drawn up professionally and legally, it is unusual for our wishes to be overturned.

What many people are unaware of is that there are strict regulations applied to a person's estate if they die intestate. You may feel safe in thinking that all will go to your spouse, or immediate next of kin when you die. However, this is not the case where the estate is valued above a certain amount (currently £75,000). Above this figure your estate will be divided up according to the law governing inheritance and it could well be that as a result, a person you would not want to benefit will in fact do so.

If you are entering a residential care home you might feel it imperative to make a will and thereby gain a greater sense of well being. It could help to allay fears that your family may have in certain areas, and also assist in addressing any resentment about your move. Your executors (it is always best to have more than one) will be aware of your views and thus able to protect your interests and those of your family. There will also be one less burden for your family to bear during what will be a sad time for them.

It is important to seek advice from a solicitor and get him or her to draw up the document for you. You will then need to make your family aware of its existence and who the executors will be, and where the document will be kept.

Further information

There are several publications which explain some of the procedures more fully and these are listed below:

Handbook for Receivers
Enduring Powers of Attorney – an explanatory booklet.

Available from The Public Trust Office free on receipt of an sae.

Leaflet AP1 *Helping Hand*, available from your local Benefits Agency.

The following are available from the Court of Protection
EP1 Notice of intention to register
EP2 Application for registration
EP3 General form of application
EP4 Application for search

The form for an EPA is *only* available from a law stationers.

How to Write a Will and Gain Probate, 5th edition, Marlene Garsia. Kogan Page, 1995.

6. Directory

The following is a list of names and addresses of organisations offering advice, information, assistance and services to the care sector of our community. These organisations can be statutory bodies, charitable institutions or private companies, covering almost every aspect of modern-day care requirements and committed to providing high-quality services.

Abbeyfield Society
53 Victoria Street
St Albans
Hertfordshire
AL1 3UW
Tel: 01727 857536

This is a federation of voluntary local societies, each having charitable status, which establish and manage family-sized houses where several elderly people live in their own bedsitting-rooms. Residents are expected to pay their own way and costs are kept to a minimum through the efforts of local volunteers.

Age Concern England (National Council on Ageing)
Astral House
1268 London Road
London
SW16 4ER
Tel: 0181 679 8000
Fax: 0181 679 6069

Age Concern is a national organisation set up in 1940 to promote the welfare of older people. The governing body is made up of representatives of over 80 national organisations and several government departments.

Age Concern England works very closely with its sister organisations in Scotland, Wales and Northern Ireland, and there are approximately 1,100 local groups in England providing a wide range of services through the help of some 180,000 volunteers.

Readers are advised to consult *The Community Care Handbook*, published by Age Concern (Ace Books). Age Concern monitors the care being carried out by various organisations.

Age Concern Cymru (Wales) (Cyngor Henoed Cymru)
1 Cathedral Road
Cardiff
CF1 9SD
Tel: 01222 371566

Age Concern Northern Ireland
6 Lower Crescent
Belfast
BT7 1NR
Tel: 01232 245729

As the law and service provision may differ from that of England and Wales, Northern Ireland readers might like to contact the above address for advice and information.

Age Concern Scotland
54A Fountainbridge
Edinburgh
EH3 9PT
Tel: 0131 228 5656

As Scottish law and service provision differs from that of England and Wales, Scottish readers might like to contact the above address for advice and information.

Age Concern Insurance Services
Garrod House
Chaldon Road
Caterham
Surrey
CR3 5YZ
Tel: 01883 346964

AllChurches Life Assurance Ltd
Beaufort House
Brunswick Road
Gloucester
GL1 1JZ
Tel: 01452 526265

A member of the 'SHIP' campaign.

Almshouse Association, The
Billingbear Lodge
Wokingham
Berkshire
RG11 5RU
Tel: 01344 52922

Details of local almshouse charities nationwide can be obtained from this association.

Alzheimer's Disease Society
Gordon House
10 Greencoat Place
London
SW1P 1PH
Tel: 0171 306 0606

This society has been set up to offer support to families and carers, and to provide information on all forms of dementia. It also runs local groups for sufferers and their relatives.

Anchor Housing Association
Anchor House
269A Banbury Road
Oxford
OX2 7HU
Tel: 01865 311511

The Association runs a Staying Put service to assist elderly home owners to improve and repair their homes for a greater degree of comfort and security.

Anchor's Staying Put team will advise on all aspects including feasibility studies, the selection of contractors and securing estimates. In the event of major structural alterations being required, the team will help in the selection of suitable architects.

The team is skilled in devising financial packages best suited to particular needs.

Anchor is also a housing trust and has a 'homes to buy or rent' service as part of its day-to-day operations.

Arthritis and Rheumatism Council, The
Copeman House
St Mary's Court
St Mary's Gate
Chesterfield
S41 7TD
Tel: 01246 558033

This organisation encourages medical research into the causes and care of arthritis and rheumatism and ensures that results of the research are made public. It also publishes a quarterly *ARC Magazine* which can be obtained on subscription.

Arthritis Care
18 Stephenson Way
London
NW1 2HD
Tel: 0171 916 1500 (counselling 1000 to 1600 hours) or Freephone Helpline 0800 289 170 (1200 to 1600 hours, Monday to Friday)

This organisation offers advice and information by highly trained counsellors, some of whom suffer from arthritis. There are more than 500 branches throughout the United Kingdom.

Association of Approved Registered Care Homes
Calthorpe House
Hagley Road
Edgbaston
Birmingham
B16 8QY
Tel: 0121 456 4401
Fax: 0121 454 0932

An association of approved registered care homes whose mission statement is:

'As professional carers we take immense care to ensure that we are sensitive to residents' needs and provide a wide range of caring and supportive services.

'By choosing our staff with care and providing induction and on-going training we ensure that our caring is individual and highly competent.

'In using quality management systems we know that our standards are consistent and reliable.'

Association of British Insurers (ABI)
51 Gresham Street
London
EC2V 7HQ
Tel: 0171 600 3333

ABI offers a free guide, *Building Insurance for Home Owners*, which contains much useful information on all forms of household insurance.

Association of Charity Officers
c/o RICS Benevolent Fund Ltd
First Floor
Tavistock House North
Tavistock Square
London
WC1H 9RJ
Tel: 0171 383 5557

The Association has about 250 members, all of whom are registered or exempt charities giving non-contributory relief and helping people from every sector of the community. The Association has no funds of its own to distribute but directs those in need of help to appropriate charities. Member organisations provide help for people in need of all ages.

The Association is staffed on a part-time basis only so it is essential that any enquiries be made in writing.

Association of Crossroads Care Attendants Schemes
See Crossroads Care.

Association of Retirement Housing Managers
50 City Way
Rochester
Kent
ME1 2AB
Tel/Fax: 01634 848639

A new organisation set up to regulate retirement housing management services by way of a code of practice. For further information contact the Secretary, Mr Ray Walker, at the above address.

Astra Housing Association
Refuge House
64–66 Stuart Street
Luton
Bedfordshire
LU1 2SW
Tel: 01582 429398

Having several schemes throughout England and Scotland, this association houses elderly people in the main. The accommodation can be independent self-contained flats, sheltered housing schemes, and residential homes where each person has their own room with washbasin and lavatory, with shared bathroom and facilities for making light snacks. Meals are provided.

Beth Johnson Housing Association Ltd, The
Three Counties House
Festival Way
Stoke-on-Trent
ST1 5PX
Tel: 01782 219200

This association operates a Staying Put service that can help with repairs and adaptations, enabling elderly people to stay in their own homes. The service can assist in obtaining grants, low-cost loans and any other benefits that might be due. As well as specifying work needed, the service will also recommend reliable builders and help in all aspects of any necessary paperwork.

Brent Reversions Services Ltd
47 Fore Street
Ivybridge
Devon
PL21 9AE
Tel: 01752 893045

British Diabetic Association
10 Queen Anne Street
London
W1M 0BD
Tel: 0171 323 1531

The Association offers help and advice to all diabetics and their families, nationwide.

British Federation of Care Home Proprietors
(BFCHP)
852 Melton Road
Thurmaston
Leicester
LE4 8BN
Tel: 0116 2640095

The BFCHP represents over 1200 homes, and membership is subject to confirmation that each home meets the Federation's standards, which are based on a national code of practice. Each home is monitored by the Federation and is visited regularly. It will supply a list of members and give general advice.

British Red Cross Society
9 Grosvenor Crescent
London
SW1X 7EJ
Tel: 0171 235 5454

The Society's services are provided mainly by volunteers from local centres, which offer home nursing, holidays and transport, and will lend equipment for frail elderly and disabled people.

British Telecom
Freephone 0800 800 150

Ask for a free copy of *BT Guide for People who are Disabled or Elderly*.

Care and Repair Ltd
Castle House
Kirtley Drive
NG7 1LD
Tel: 0115 979 9091

London Office
168–172 Old Street
London
EC1V 9BP
Tel: 0171 336 7719

This society was established by Shelter and the Housing Associations Charitable Trust to develop and support Care and Repair projects. In 1991 Care and Repair Ltd was chosen by government to be the national co-ordinating body for home improvement agencies.

Other offices are situated as follows:

Care and Repair
Scottish Homes
Mercantile Chambers
53 Bothwell Street
Glasgow
G2 6TS
Tel: 0141 248 7177

Care and Repair Cymru
Norbury House
Norbury Road
Fairwater
Cardiff
CF5 3AS
Tel: 01222 576286

Carers' National Association
20–25 Glasshouse Yard
London EC1A 4JS
Tel: 0171 490 8818
Adviceline: 0171 490 8898 (1300–1600 weekdays)

London Region
5 Chalton Street
London NW1 1JD
Tel: 0171 383 3460

Scotland
11 Queens Crescent
Glasgow G4 9AS
Tel: 0141 333 9495

NW Yorkshire and Humberside Region
Chalton House
Salem Church
36 Hunslet Road
Leeds LS10 1JN
Tel: 0532 449228

The Association provides information and support for people caring for sick, disabled or frail elderly relatives or friends. A range of free leaflets is available.

Caresearch
c/o United Response
162–164 Upper Richmond Road
London
SW15 2SL
Tel: 0181 780 9596

The Caresearch database contains information on residential care throughout Britain. There is a fee payable for each search.

Carlyle Life Assurance Co Ltd
21 Windsor Place
Cardiff
CF1 3BY
Tel: 01222 371726

A member of the 'SHIP' campaign; PIA registered.

Castle Rock Housing Association Ltd
2 Wishaw Terrace
Meadowbank
Edinburgh
EH7 6AF
Tel: 0131 652 0152

A non-profit organisation specialising in providing purpose-built sheltered and amenity housing for rent and sale.

Cavendish Home Reversions Ltd
(Incorporating Age Alliance)
6 Allerton Hill
Leeds
LS7 3QD
Tel: 01532 370666

Centre for Accessible Environments
Nutmeg House
60 Gainsford Street
London
SE1 2NY
Tel: 0171 357 8182

This national voluntary organisation is concerned with improving the design of the built environment to accommodate the needs of all users, including the elderly and disabled.

Charity Search
25 Portview Road
Avonmouth
Bristol
BS11 9LD
Tel: 0117 982 4060

A charity which provides free advice for elderly people and puts them in touch with other charities which may be able to assist with funds for top-up of fees in residential or nursing homes, or with extra costs at home.

Church of Ireland Housing Association (NI) Ltd
74 Dublin Road
Belfast
BT2 7HP
Tel: 01232 242130

This charity provides housing for the elderly throughout Northern Ireland, catering for the more active person as well as those needing sheltered care. Allocations are made on the basis of a points system.

Continence Foundation
2 Doughty Street
London
WC1N 2PH

For general information and advice, write to this address.

Continence Foundation Helpline
The Dene Centre
Castles Farm Road
Newcastle upon Tyne
NE3 1PH
Tel: 0191 213 0050 (Monday to Friday, 1400 to 1900 hours)

For general information and advice.

Counsel and Care for the Elderly
Twyman House
16 Bonny Street
London
NW1 9PG
Tel: 0171 485 1566 (1030 to 1600 hours only)

This registered charity provides a nationwide service and free advice and information service for older people, their carers and professional carers each year. Enquiries are dealt with by letter or telephone and, where necessary, referred to more specific organisations. A comprehensive list of fact sheets is available on request.

Grants. Counsel and Care administer several trust funds and it is possible, subject to financial resources, for single payment grants to be made to individuals.

Home visits. Advice workers visit registered private and voluntary residential care and nursing homes in the Greater London area every 12 to 18 months. As a result of the information gathered, they are able to offer suggestions and advice in respect of homes most suited to specific needs.

Country Houses Association Ltd
41 Kingsway
London
WC2B 6UB
Tel: 0171 836 1624

This association is a registered charity and has two main objectives:

- To save, for the benefit of the nation, houses of historic importance, architectural interest, or of beauty which may otherwise decay through inability of individual owners to keep them maintained.
- To create within the houses apartments for letting as residential accommodation.

Crossroads Care
10 Regent Place
Rugby
Warwickshire
CV21 2PN
Tel: 01788 573653

This organisation has more than 200 schemes throughout the UK which aim to offer respite to carers.

Cruse – Bereavement Care
Cruse House
126 Sheen Road
Richmond
Surrey
TW9 1UR
Tel: 0181 940 4818
0181 332 7227 Bereavement line, Monday to Friday 0930 to 1700 hours.

This organisation offers a counselling service for bereaved people throughout the country.

CSV Volunteer Programme
237 Pentonville Road
London
N1 9NJ
Tel: 0171 278 6601

This national organisation places young people to assist full time as Community Service Volunteers (CSVs), for between 4 and 12 months. They must be provided with accommodation, food, pocket money and travel expenses, and supervised regularly by a third party. An annual fee is payable to CSV.
   For more information contact the above address or:

CSV Scotland
236 Clyde Street
Glasgow
G1 4JH
Tel: 0141 204 1681

Department of Social Security (DSS)

The welfare rights and benefits section of the DSS is called the Benefits Agency.
Freephone 0800 666 555 offers information and general advice on benefits. Also see your local telephone directory.

Derwent Housing Association Ltd
Phoenix Street
Derby
DE1 2ER
Tel: 01332 46477

A non-profit association registered with the Housing Corporation and the Registrar of Friendly Societies, its objectives are to provide accommodation for those in need.

Disabled Housing Trust
Norfolk Lodge
Oakenfield
Burgess Hill
West Sussex
RH15 8SJ
Tel: 01444 239123

A registered national charity, the Trust provides specialist housing for physically handicapped people, either as sheltered housing or residential accommodation.

Disabled Living Centres Council
The Basement
2 Doughty Street
London WC1N 2PH
Tel: 0171 404 6875

Lower Ground Floor
Twyman House
16 Bonny Street
London NW1 9PG
Tel: 0171 485 1566 (1000 to 1600 hours)

Public Trust Office
Protection Division
Stewart House
24 Kingsway
London WC2B 6JX
Tel: 0171 269 7157/7358/7317

10 Regent Place
Rugby
Warwickshire CV21 2PN
Tel: 01788 573653

286 Camden Road
London N7 0BJ
Tel: 0171 700 1707

Also listed in telephone directories or in *Yellow Pages* under

'Counselling and Advice'. They can tell you your nearest Disabled Living Centre where you can see and try out aids and equipment.

Disabled Living Foundation
380–384 Harrow Road
London
W9 2HU
Tel: 0171 289 6111 (Monday to Friday, 1000 to 1600 hours)

This is a national charity specialising in advice and up-to-date information on the many and varied aspects of living with a disability. It operates an Enquiry Service and has specific details about equipment designed to assist disabled and elderly people.

Elderly Accommodation Counsel
46A Chiswick High Road
London
W4 1SZ
Tel: 0181 742 1182
     0181 995 8320
Fax: 0181 995 7714

The objectives of this charity are: to provide information and advice on all forms of accommodation suitable to meet the needs of retired and elderly people; and to give advice on possible sources of top-up funding.

EAC have a national register of all types of accommodation in the voluntary and private sectors including nursing homes, terminal hospices, sheltered housing and sheltered accommodation. A simple questionnaire is required to get computer print-outs about suitable accommodation. A fee of £5.00 is charged for this service, but in cases of extreme need this can be waived.

English Churches Housing Group
Sutherland House
70–78 West Hendon Broadway
London
NW9 7BT
Tel: 0181 203 9233
Fax: 0181 203 0092

The Group works in partnership with local communities to provide quality homes with appropriate care and support services, accessible to those in need. As a Christian-based housing association, it provides emergency and general needs housing, supported housing, and sheltered accommodation. Regional offices manage homes for people of all ages, from all sections of the community. ECHG aims to promote social justice in housing and remains committed to equality of opportunity.

ECHG also operates a care arm called Heritage Care.

English Courtyard Association
8 Holland Street
London
W8 4LT
Tel: 0171 937 4511

The Association is a non-profit organisation providing specialised luxury accommodation for elderly retired people. The cottages and flats are developed along the lines of the traditional courtyard plan of almshouses.

The properties are usually sold on long leases of 150 years and the occupier, though not necessarily the owner, must be of retirement age.

Family Welfare Association
501–505 Kingsland Road
London
E8 4AU
Tel: 0171 254 6251

This association offers housing for elderly people in almshouses.

Federation of Private Residents Associations Ltd
62 Bayswater Road
London
W2 3PS
Tel: 0171 402 1581

This is a co-ordinating body for tenants' and residents' associations in England and Wales. It provides an information pack on how to form a tenants' or leaseholders' association for people living in flats, maisonettes or in converted properties. It also advises on tenants' rights and landlords' obligations under the terms of housing legislation.

Financial Intermediaries, Managers and Brokers Regulatory Association (FIMBRA)
Hertsmere House
Hertsmere Road
London
E14 4AB
Tel: 0171 538 8860
       0171 895 1229
Fax: 0171 895 8579

The regulatory body for independent financial advisers. However, as from October 1995 this organisation will be incorporated within the Personal Investment Authority. Individuals currently registered with FIMBRA are not necessarily required to register with the PIA, but they are required to register with a regulatory body.

Five Counties Housing Association Ltd
Three Counties House
Festival Way
Stoke-on-Trent
ST1 5PX
Tel: 01782 219200

A sister association to the Beth Johnson Housing Association, Five Counties has developed purpose-built bungalows and apartments at 70 per cent of cost for elderly home buyers.

Fold Housing Association
3 Redburn Square
Holywood
Co Down
BT18 9HZ
Tel: 01232 428314

This association specialises in building sheltered housing for the elderly throughout Northern Ireland.

Friends of the Elderly and Gentlefolk's Help
42 Ebury Street
London
SW1W 0LZ
Tel: 0171 730 8263

Operates 12 homes, some of which have nursing wings where short- or long-stay patients may reside. Generally, residents are asked to furnish their own rooms, including curtains, carpets and bedding. Fees are based upon residents' income and capital, and residents are not required to pay more than they can afford.

Grace
35 Walnut Tree Close
Guildford
Surrey
GU1 4UL
Tel: 01483 304354

This organisation matches people's requirements with its database to produce a short-list of possible homes. Their representatives visit homes on their list once a year, and the area covered is England south of Birmingham. A fee is charged for their service.

Guardian Housing Association Ltd
Anchor House
269A Banbury Road
Oxford
OX2 7HU
Tel: 01865 311711

Working in association with Anchor Housing Association and Housing Trust, Guardian provides and manages sheltered accommodation for older people able to purchase their own property. Offering a range of properties from shared ownership to outright ownership, it currently manages in excess of 5000 properties throughout England.

Guild of Aid for Gentlepeople
10 St Christopher's Place
London
W1M 6HY
Tel: 0171 935 0641

Confidential assistance given to persons of gentle birth or good education who, by reason of ill health, old age, illness or other disability are unable to work.

Guinness Trust, The
17 Mendy Street
High Wycombe
Buckinghamshire
HP11 2NZ
Tel: 01494 535823

This organisation provides warden-supervised flats for elderly people within the Trust's larger housing projects.

Hanover Housing Association
Hanover House
18 The Avenue
Egham
Surrey
TW20 9AB
Tel: 01784 438361

Provides and manages accommodation for rent to older people throughout England and Wales. The properties, usually self-contained one-bedroomed dwellings, are supervised by resident wardens; all dwellings are connected to the warden's home by a communication system.

Its office in Scotland is at:

36 Albany Street
Edinburgh
EH1 3QH
Tel: 0131 557 0598

Help the Aged
St James's Walk
Clerkenwell Green
London
EC1R 0BE
Tel: 0171 253 0253
Fax: 0171 895 1407

Help the Aged is a national charity, primarily fundraising, which gives grants to community-based projects such as day centres, minibuses, community alarms and hospices. It also offers services directly to the elderly and their carers such as SeniorLine (0800 289 404), a free national information service for the elderly, their relatives, carers and friends. Advice workers are able to give general information on a variety of subjects, including: welfare and disability benefits; health; housing; support for carers; mobility; community alarms; sources of local help; other voluntary organisations.

All calls to SeniorLine are treated in the strictest confidence and the line is open Monday to Friday, 1000 to 1600 hours.

The organisation publishes a range of free advice leaflets on such subjects as money, home safety and health; these leaflets can be obtained by writing to the Information Department and enclosing a 9″ × 6″ stamped, self-addressed envelope.

Help the Aged also runs residential homes, extra-sheltered housing, sheltered housing and a gifted housing scheme.

Heritage Housing Ltd
36 Albany Street
Edinburgh
EH1 3QH
Tel: 0131 557 0598

A non-profit housing association formed by Hanover (Scotland) Housing Association to develop and build sheltered housing for sale to the elderly. It is totally independent of Hanover.

Hinton and Wild (Home Plans) Ltd
374–378 Ewell Road
Surbiton
Surrey
KT6 7BB
Tel: 0181 390 8166

Acts as the co-ordinating secretary for the 'SHIP' campaign.

Holiday Care Service
2 Old Bank Chambers
Station Road
Horley
Surrey
RH6 9HW
Tel: 01293 774535
Minicom: 01293 776943

An information service for people who are elderly or disabled, single parents or carers and have severe financial pressures.

Home and Capital Trust Ltd
31 Goldington Road
Bedford
MK40 3LH
Tel: 01234 340511

A member of the 'SHIP' campaign.

Homelife/Distressed Gentlefolk's Aid Association
Vicarage Gate House
Vicarage Gate
London
W8 4AQ
Tel: 0171 229 9341
Fax: 0171 792 9828

The main objective of this organisation is to enable people to stay in their own homes; however it also helps by top-up of residential home fees. Its services are offered to those of British or Irish nationality and of a professional or similar background.

Homes (Housing Organisations Mobility and Exchange Services)
26 Chapter Street
London
SW1P 4ND
Tel: 0171 233 7077
Fax: 0171 976 6947

The aim of this organisation is to help local authorities and housing association tenants to move house.

Hospice Information Service
St Christopher's Hospice
51–59 Lawrie Park Road
London
SE26 6DZ
Tel: 0181 778 9252

This organisation offers information to the public and health care professionals about the work of the hospice movement. It produces a directory of UK hospices, and written or telephone enquiries are welcomed.

Housing Associations Charitable Trust (HACT)
3rd Floor
Yeoman House
168–172 Old Street
London
EC1V 9BP
Tel: 0171 336 7969
Fax: 0171 336 7721

This is a grant-making trust which supports voluntary housing organisations throughout the UK. Its current priorities include assisting small organisations, black, ethnic minority and refugee groups.

Housing Corporation, The
149 Tottenham Court Road
London
W1P 0BN
Tel: 0171 393 2000
Fax: 0171 393 2111

The Corporation's prime function is to promote, register and supervise 2,300 registered housing associations in England. It provides a comprehensive and responsive service to housing associations and to those people and agencies who deal with them. It also distributes government funds as grants to projects carried out by registered housing associations.

Contact the above address for information about its area offices.

Investment Property Reversions Ltd
34 Hillcrest Road
Purley
Surrey
CR8 2JE
Tel: 0181 645 9444

James Butcher Housing Association
James Butcher House
39 High Street
Theale
Reading
RG7 5AH
Tel: 01734 323434

A charitable association providing rented accommodation mainly for the elderly in the counties of Berkshire, Buckinghamshire, Gloucestershire, Hampshire, Oxfordshire, Surrey, Sussex and Wiltshire.

Jephson Homes Housing Association Ltd
Jephson House
Blackdown
Leamington Spa
Warwickshire
CV32 6RE
Tel: 01926 339311

Formed to provide homes for the elderly, the Association now builds and manages new homes for letting, leasing, sale and shared ownership.

Jewish Care
Stuart Young House
221 Golders Green Road
London
NW11 9DQ
Tel: 0181 458 3282
Fax: 0181 731 8307

This organisation provides services and help to elderly, mentally ill, visually impaired and physically disabled people and their families.

Kirk Care Housing Association Ltd
3 Forres Street
Edinburgh
EH3 6BJ
Tel: 0131 225 7246

533 Baltic Chambers
50 Wellington Street
Glasgow
G2 6HJ
Tel: 0141 221 3445

58–60 Church Street
Inverness
Tel: 01463 240344

Kirk Care is a non-profit company providing sheltered housing for the elderly in Scotland. The Association is keen to develop 'continuing care' so that people who become frail need not be moved into residential care.

Lautro Ltd (LAUTRO)
103 New Oxford Street
London
WC1A 1QH
Tel: 0171 379 0444

The Life Assurance and Unit Trust Regulatory Organisation is responsible for the regulation of the retail marketing of life assurances and unit trusts by life companies, friendly societies and authorised unit trusts.

After October 1995 LAUTRO will be incorporated within the Personal Investment Authority (PIA). Companies already registered with LAUTRO are not necessarily required to register with PIA but they are required to register with a 'regulatory body'. Companies who provide lump-sum payments are not required to register.

Merseyside Improved Homes
Wavertree Road
Liverpool
L7 1PH
Tel: 0151 709 9375

This housing association provides almost 17,000 homes in the Merseyside area, with the major proportion being for elderly people.

Methodist Homes for the Aged
Epworth House
Stuart Street
Derby
DE1 2EQ
Tel: 01332 296200

This organisation runs 22 sheltered housing schemes throughout the UK for elderly people (not necessarily Methodists).

National Association of Estate Agents
Arbon House
21 Jury Street
Warwick
CV34 4EH
Tel: 01926 496800

National Bed Line
J and F House
164 Merton Road
London
SW19 1EG
Tel: 0181 540 5455

A free 24-hour information service to help people find places in private and voluntary residential and nursing homes. The service also covers private hospitals, hospices, and most local authority residential homes.

National Care Homes Association
5 Bloomsbury Place
London
WC1A 2QA
Tel: 0171 436 1871
Fax: 0171 436 1193

This is a confederation of local associations of private care homes. The NCHA operates a code of conduct which all members are required to observe. There is also a residents' charter which outlines what level of service is due to residents. Twenty-five specific areas are covered within this charter.

National Federation of Housing Associations
175 Gray's Inn Road
London
WC1X 8UP
Tel: 0171 278 6571
Fax: 0171 955 5696

This is the representative body for housing associations in England, providing information for its members and representing their interests to government, local authorities and other bodies. The NFHA has ten regional offices in England. Housing associations in Scotland, Wales and Northern Ireland have their own federations, as follows:

Northern Ireland Federation of Housing Associations
88 Clifton Street
Belfast
BT13 1AB
Tel: 01232 230446

Scottish Federation of Housing Associations
40 Castle Street North
Edinburgh
EH2 3BN
Tel: 0131 226 6777

Welsh Federation of Housing Associations
Norbury House
Norbury Road
Fairwater
Cardiff
CF5 3AS
Tel: 01222 555022

National House Building Council
Buildmark House
Chiltern Avenue
Amersham
Buckinghamshire
HP6 5AP
Tel: 01494 434477
Fax: 01494 728521

Operates the Sheltered Housing Code which is obligatory to all its members.

National Housing Trust Ltd
(Development Arm of Nationwide Building Society)
Moulton Park
Northampton
NN3 1NL
Tel: 01604 794189

The Trust has a variety of sheltered retirement homes for sale.

New Homes Marketing Board
82 New Cavendish Street
London
W1M 8AD

This organisation can supply a list of developers engaged in building sheltered housing. Initial enquiries in writing, please.

North British Housing Association Group
11th Floor
Unicentre
Lords Walk
Preston
PR1 1DP
Tel: 01772 24441

4 The Pavilions
Portway
Preston
PR2 2YB
Tel: 01772 897200

This non-profit organisation is one of the leading associations in the UK with over 30,000 homes under its management. It is involved in the provision of care and support facilities for older people as well as providing good quality, well managed accommodation for rent or sale. It also operates a Staying Put scheme in the Blackburn area.

Northern Counties Homes
Princes Building
Oxford Court
Oxford Street
Manchester
M2 3WQ
Tel: 0161 228 3388
     0161 228 3333 (24 hours)

As part of the Northern Counties Housing Association Ltd, this organisation specialises in the sale of sheltered housing on long leases.

Northern Counties Housing Association Ltd
Princes Building
15 Oxford Court
Oxford Street
Manchester
M2 3WQ
Tel: 0161 228 3388

This association specialises in sheltered housing schemes for sale or rent, with resident wardens and communal facilities, throughout the north of England.

Northern Ireland Co-ownership Housing Association Ltd
Murray House
Murray Street
Belfast
BT1 6DN
Tel: 01232 327276

This association specialises in part-ownership schemes whereby the purchaser buys a 50 per cent stake in a house and pays rent for the balance. Only properties with an asking price of less than £36,000 are considered.

Northern Ireland and Housing Executive
The Housing Centre
2 Adelaide Street
Belfast
BT2 8PB
Tel: 01232 240588

Specialises in helping people to improve, repair or adapt their homes and, where necessary, to move to a more suitable environment.

North Housing
Ridley House
Regent Centre
Newcastle upon Tyne
NE3 3JE
Tel: 0191 285 0311

This organisation provides sheltered housing for older people to rent in the north east, north west, south east and the east Midlands.

Nursing Home Fees Agency
Old Bank House
95 London Road
Oxford
OX3 9AE
Tel: 01865 750665

This agency offers information on welfare benefits entitlement and independent financial advice on investment of capital.

Office of Fair Trading
Field House
15–25 Bream's Buildings
London
EC4A 1PR
Tel: 0171 242 2858

Publishes the free leaflet, *Home Improvements*, which carries comprehensive advice on all aspects of arranging home improvements, including a list of relevant trade and professional organisations that operate a code of practice.

Orbit Housing Association
44–45 Queens Road
Coventry
West Midlands
CV1 3EH
Tel: 01203 632231

This association operates in London and from the following regional offices:

Midlands Region
5–7 Dormer Place
Leamington Spa
Warwickshire
CV32 5AA
Tel: 01926 32255

London and Home Counties Region
23 Ewell Road
Cheam
Surrey
SM3 8DD
Tel: 0181 661 9921

Eastern Region
14 St Matthew's Road
Norwich
NR1 1SP
Tel: 01603 614348

Western Region
5 Beaufort Park
Woodlands
Almondsbury
Bristol
BS12 4NE
Tel: 0117 9617666

Orbit Spa Housing Association Ltd
44–45 Queens Road
Coventry
West Midlands
CV1 3EH
Tel: 01203 632231

This is the charitable arm of the Orbit Housing Association.

Parkinson's Disease Society of the UK
22 Upper Woburn Place
London
WC1H 0RA
Tel: 0171 383 3513
Helpline: 0171 388 5798 (Monday to Friday, 1000 to 1600 hours)

The society provides information and advice for people caring for someone with Parkinson's disease. It has many local branches.

Patients Association
18 Victoria Park Square
Bethnal Green
London
E2 9PF
Tel: 0181 981 5676 (Monday to Friday, 0930 to 1730)
　　 0181 981 5695 (Monday to Friday, 0930 to 1730)

This association offers advice to patients and carers on patients' rights and complaints procedures and access to health services or specific self-help groups.

Personal Investment Authority (PIA)
3–4 Royal Exchange Buildings
London
EC3V 3NL
Tel: 0171 929 0072

A new regulatory body which came into effect in July 1994. It incorporates FIMBRA and LAUTRO, both of which will cease to exist after October 1995.

Members of the public will now have just one body to register complaints with, and an added bonus is access to the PIA Ombudsman.

Presbyterian Housing Association (NI) Ltd
Lowry House
27 Hampton Park
Belfast
BT8 4AX
Tel: 01232 491851

The main objective of the Association is to provide sheltered housing to elderly people throughout Northern Ireland regardless of their religious beliefs.

Quaker Social Responsibility and Education
Friends House
Euston Road
London
NW1 2BJ
Tel: 0171 387 3601

A list, 'Accommodation for Elderly People under Quaker Auspices', is available from the above address.

RADAR (The Royal Association for Disability and Rehabilitation
12 City Forum
250 City Road
London
EC1V 8AF
Tel: 0171 250 3222

Offers advice and information to Britain's disabled people, their families and carers.

Regentsmead Group
140 High Street
Edgware
Middlesex
HA8 7LW
Tel: 0181 951 1996

Registered Nursing Homes Association
Calthorpe House
Hagley Road
Edgbaston
Birmingham
B16 8QY
Tel: 0121 454 2511

With more than 1,200 registered nursing homes, members of this association operate a rigorous standards policy. The sign of the Blue Cross indicates that an establishment meets these standards.

Relatives Association
5 Tavistock Place
London
WC1H 9SS
Tel: 0171 916 6055

This is an organisation dedicated to improving residential and nursing home care for the elderly by involving their relatives.

Residential Home Reversions Ltd
154A Brighton Road
Widewater
Lancing
Sussex
BN15 8LL
Tel: 01903 761244

Retirement Lease Housing Association
19 Eggar's Court
St George's Road East
Aldershot
Hampshire
GU12 4LN
Tel: 01252 318181

An association that provides and manages housing schemes

(flats and bungalows) specially designed for active elderly owner occupiers.

Royal Air Forces Association
Portland Road
Malvern
Worcestershire
WR14 2TA
Tel: 01684 892505

This association works closely with the Royal Air Force Benevolent Fund.

Royal British Legion Housing Association Ltd
PO Box 32
St John's Road
Penn
High Wycombe
Buckinghamshire
HP10 8JF
Tel: 0149 481 3771

This association, while having a direct responsibility to ex-service people, will consider applications from others needing sheltered housing or care.

Royal National Institute for the Blind (RNIB)
224 Great Portland Street
London
W1N 6AA
Tel: 0171 388 1266

Provides information and advice for those with visual disabilities.

Royal United Kingdom Beneficent Association (RUKBA)
6 Avonmore Road
London
W14 8RL
Tel: 0171 602 6274
Fax: 0171 371 1807

The Association offers help to elderly professional people or those from a similar background. It assists and encourages these people to remain in their own homes, and it also provides residential and nursing homes for the frail and sick.

Saga Services Ltd
The Saga Building
Middleburg Square
Folkestone
Kent
CT20 1AZ
Tel: 01303 857526
Freephone: 0800 414525

Offers insurance to people aged 55 or over with a 'Homecare Plan' for buildings and contents.

SHAC (The London Housing Aid Centre)
189A Old Brompton Road
London
SW5 0AR
Tel: 0171 373 7276

SHAC is a registered charity which provides a wide range of help and advice on all housing matters throughout London.

Sheltered Housing Advisory and Conciliation Service
Walkden House
3–10 Melton Street
London
NW1 2EJ
Tel: 0171 383 2006

This organisation offers an arbitration service in the event of disputes arising from the sale and purchase of sheltered housing.

Sheltered Housing Owners Confederation of Scotland
107–173 Comley Bank Road
Edinburgh
EH4 1DH
Tel: 0131 343 6100

This organisation was set up to safeguard the welfare of elderly owners of sheltered housing in Scotland. It is also affiliated with Age Concern Scotland.

Sheltered Housing Services Ltd
8–9 Abbey Parade
North Circular Road
London
W5 1EE
Tel: 0181 997 9313

This is an independent company offering a specialist service to anyone seeking to purchase a retirement home. A small fee is required for its list of nationwide projects.

Shelter – National Campaign for Homeless People
88 Old Street
London
EC1V 9HU
Tel: 0171 253 0202

Shelter provides free and confidential advice through a network of Housing Aid Centres to anyone experiencing housing problems.

SHIP Campaign
Hinton and Wild (Home Plans) Ltd
374 Ewell Road
Surbiton
Surrey
KT6 7BB
Tel: 0181 390 8166

Safe Home Income Plan. See page 77.

Shires Housing Association Ltd, The
Three Counties House
Festival Way
Stoke-on-Trent
ST1 5PX
Tel: 01782 219200

(See Five Counties Housing Association Ltd.)

Sovereign Reversions Plc
c/o Johnson Fry PLC
20 Regent Street
London
SW1Y 4PZ
Tel: 0171 321 0220

Special Interest Group – Adult Placement Schemes
Social Services Department
The Council House
Solihull
West Midlands
B91 3QY
Tel: 0121 704 6743

Stalwart Assurance Company Ltd
Stalwart House
142 South Street
Dorking
Surrey
RH4 2EU
Tel: 01306 876581
Freephone: 0800 378921

A member of the 'SHIP' campaign and PIA registered.

Stroke Association
CHSA House
123–127 Whitecross Street
London
EC1Y 8JJ
Tel: 0171 490 7999

Lists available about stroke support and rehabilitation groups. Also offers stroke sufferers and their families counselling and welfare services.

The Sutton Housing Trust
Sutton Court
Tring
Hertfordshire
HP23 5BB
Tel: 01442 891100

The Trust is a registered housing association which provides quality rented accommodation with resident managers and maintenance staff for people on low incomes and in housing need.

United Kingdom Home Care Association
c/o 22 Southway
Carshalton
Surrey
SM5 4HW
Tel: 0181 770 3658

An association of private home care agencies that operate its code of practice.

Women's Royal Voluntary Service (WRVS) Trust
233–244 Stockwell Road
London
SW9 9SP
Tel: 0171 416 0146

WRVS Residential Care for the Elderly.
WRVS All-Day and Luncheon Clubs for the Elderly.

Further information concerning the work of WRVS can be obtained from the Secretary, WRVS Trustees Limited at the above address.

The WRVS is actively engaged in the meals-on-wheels service which is usually activated through its local branches. It also offers other support facilities for elderly people and their carers.

Bibliography

The Ageing Parent Handbook 1994, Belinda Hadden. Thorsons

Charities Digest 1994. The Family Welfare Association

Directory for Older People, compiled by Ann Darnborough and Derek Kinrade. Harvester Wheatsheaf in association with Age Concern

A Guide to Grants for Individuals in Need, edited by David Casson and Paul Brown. Directory of Social Change

Health and Safety in Residential Care Homes. HSE Books

Social Services Year Book 1994. Longman Information and Reference

Staying at Home: Helping Elderly People, Anthea Tinker. HMSO

Magazines and journals

Retirement Homes and Finance (monthly)
Selwood Press Ltd
Unit 1, Raans Road
Amersham
Buckinghamshire
HP6 6LX
Tel: 0494 432433

Retirement Planning and Living (monthly)
Community Media Avon Ltd
1 City Business Park
Bristol
BS5 0SP
Tel: 0117 9555550

List of Advertisers

Index